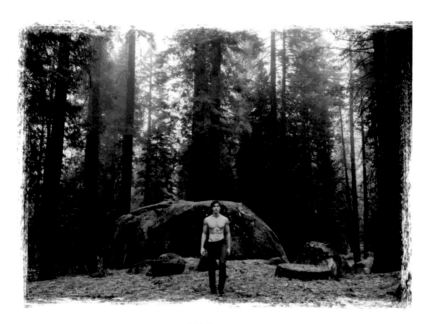

*Welcome.*

Braeden Baade

# The Nature Physique

Written by:

Braeden Baade

Edited by:

Marcella Kotlarz

Formatted by:

Damien Benoit-Ledoux

http://www.NaturePhysiqueFitness.com

*To all who cherish a healthy lifestyle.*

Braeden Baade

# Foreword

I want my readers to understand that *The Nature Physique* plan is not just an exercise regimen; it's a way of life. This way of life includes notions such as doing all you can to think positively, living in the moment, living graciously, and always treating others with kindness. I simply cannot emphasize enough that the combination of these components form a fulfilling life.

As you absorb the content of this book, and begin to perform the variety of exercises, be mindful to incorporate a state of gratitude and inner-peace. Become one with mother nature and become one with your *nature physique.*

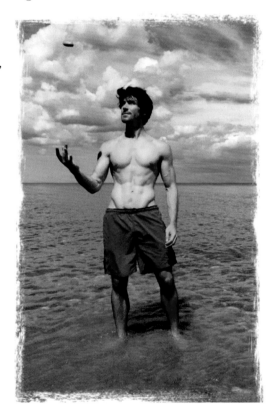

Evolve...

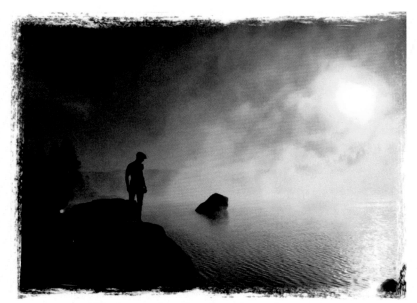

*"Early to bed and early to rise makes a man healthy, wealthy, and wise."*

*— Benjamin Franklin*

# Introduction

What is this... "nature physique?" Well, let me describe it to you in the simplest way possible. It's the call of the wild or the physical appearance that glorious mother nature intended for every human to have. Much of our species would have maintained this lean, solid build if we were still running wild, hunting and consuming a protein rich diet.

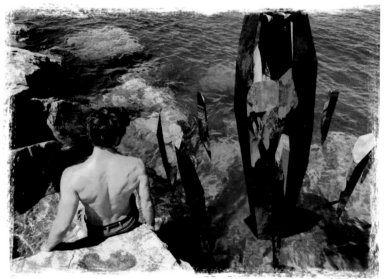

The *nature physique* is all about returning to the roots of our ancestors, before silly, anabolic supplement companies, corny infomercials, and sometimes obnoxious (and unnecessary) corporate gym franchises came into play. These enterprises are often run by brain-washing, greedy, manipulative capitalistic intentions. Many of those dietary supplements that you often browse over in a supplement shop (I won't name any names but I'm certain that you can think of some) aren't even evaluated by the FDA (Food and Drug Administration). How can one even begin to fathom the variety of long term side effects the human body may endure from these chemicals? You can't, but at least one thing is certain; the contents of your wallet will expose some damaging side effects!

I will say that if you've been searching far and wide for that "perfect" formula that will transform you into a beefed-up, monstrous, ape-like-creature... you've most definitely stumbled upon the wrong piece of literature. If you're looking for the secret to gaining a bulging abdominal eight-pack with veins that look as though they're moments away from bursting through an orange and greasy fake tan... yes, you've come to the right place! Just kidding. But all joking aside, if you have an appetite for knowledge about how to simplify and overcome the modern-day obstacles to becoming fit, healthy, and feeling great, this book will help get you on the right path.

I learned to harness my own *nature physique* while spending a couple of years working as a model in the fashion industry. Now, if you've ever considered this subject, it's important to keep in mind that modeling for the fitness industry and modeling for the fashion industry are two completely different things. Put simply, one requires you to look like a meat-head, while the other requires you to look naturally toned and chiseled, without appearing as though you spend every waking moment in the gym. You can probably guess which is which. The fashion industry has a desire for men who look buff when shirtless, but are still small enough to fit into and show off the latest designer suit in a 38 or 40 jacket size. In the fashion industry, the allure seems to come from the assumption that the model is just naturally gifted. In a career where your competition is scrambling around to obtain that physique, as well as maintain it, you need to figure out what formula works for you. I had difficulty with this at first.

Before moving to New York and trying my hand at the 'modeling' business, I had recently graduated from university, where I played lacrosse on a competitive collegiate level. It was a necessity for me to have the extra muscle packed on just so I could survive the physicality of the sport, both against other athletes on the field as well as to withstand the rigorous training program off the field. However, rather inconveniently for me, a bulky build has no place in the world of fashion, which forced me to re-evaluate my exercise and nutrition plans. I soon realized that my new approach may be quite appealing and useful to the general population.

I intended for this book to be overflowing with positive life-force. I wanted it to help those who lack the time and simply don't want to spend their hard-earned money on a personal trainer. I want to lay it out for you; if you're looking to uncover your *nature physique*, you don't need an expensive personal trainer!

Of course, we all know there are a variety of body-types out there, each of which require different levels of maintenance. The best part about *nature physique* training is that whether you feel you're overly-thin or overly-heavy, the regime is identical.

I've witnessed many people morph their appearance, strength, and overall health while training under my regimen three to four times per week, with sessions lasting no longer than 40 minutes. I've watched those same people receive compliments on their progress from their friends who had no clue they were undertaking any sort of new routine. That's a rewarding feeling.

It's important to note that I don't hold personal training sessions anymore and haven't for a few years now. In fact, I can't even claim that I work as a fitness industry professional during the time I'm writing this book. However, not a day goes by where I haven't continued to work on my craft, mentally recording what works for myself and retaining what worked for my clientele.

As you work your way through this book, a new world of fitness-simplicity shall manifest itself to you. Mother Nature intended for you to discover your *nature physique* and run wild with it, honoring the biological shell with which you were gifted.

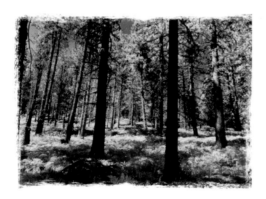

# Author's Note

If at any point you feel that the following chapters fail to hold your interest, I'd like to give the option to skip over them and immediately dive into the instructional portions of this book. Many readers may find the proceeding information irrelevant but I did feel an obligation to elaborate a bit on the origin of this book and my personal journey to discovering my *nature physique.*

# Disclaimer

All of the information and opinions expressed in *The Nature Physique* are entirely my own and based upon my own personal perspective and experiences. I do not purport that this information is based on any accurate, current or valid scientific knowledge and as such the author will not be liable for any losses, injuries or damages arising from its display or use. Please use your own discretion when exercising and consult your health-care provider if you feel any discomfort when performing any of the exercises.

# Chapter 1 – A Bit About Me

If you have managed to get this far, you're probably wondering who I am exactly? How about I start off by re-assuring you that I do at least have professional fitness credibility attached to my name. As far as fitness training and nutrition consultation goes, I became licensed through ACSM (the American College of Sports Medicine) back in 2011, but I will elaborate more on that later.

Lake Bluff, Illinois is where I was raised. In 2012 this heavenly place was ranked number 4 (out of 15) on *Coastal Living's* "America's Happiest Seaside Towns". I had an idyllic childhood filled with love

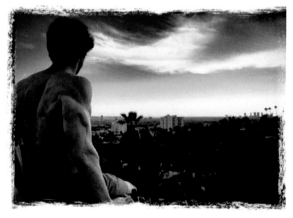

and I feel incredibly lucky to have such a wonderful, supportive family who have encouraged me to be the best version of myself.

My dad was a major motivating factor in the creation of this book. He is without a doubt the hardest worker I know on both a mental and physical level. As both a well-known economics professor and professional sports economics consultant, the guy takes on an extremely demanding work load. However, he never neglects an opportunity to take care of his body by squeezing in time for exercise. Whether waking up extra early to attend the local gym, or performing a calisthenics routine on the floor while watching his favorite Green Bay Packers compete, he's always up for the chance to strive for better physical shape. I now do my best to mimic that way of life.

There was always a big emphasis on sports while growing up within my household, whether it was participating or spectating, sports were a popular topic of discussion. Beginning at an early age I was gently encouraged to participate in basketball, baseball, tennis, and whatever other leagues, camps, and clinics were offered by the park district. As far as I can remember I started off strong, feeling faster, more coordinated, and overall more athletic than most children in my age group. But, unfortunately, that did not last very long as my growth came to a halt for quite some time. This, and I'm assuming is the case for so many others, was a major blow to my confidence. I don't recall that I completely caught up to speed until around my junior year of high school, which was when I took keen interest in the great sport of lacrosse.

Because I started playing lacrosse so late in my high school career, I'm sure you can imagine I had a lot of catching up to do. Luckily, I was able to round up both the discipline and determination needed to go on and play college ball at NCAA Division II, Saint Leo University, located on the outskirts of Tampa, Florida. With the privilege of being able to play a college sport, and the fierce competition that comes along with that, I decided I was going to test my limits as to how strong I could become and how much muscle mass/weight I could pack on along with it.

I can't say I remember exactly what my "gains" were when I reached my peak but I will estimate at the early age of 18, I was around 6 feet and weighed about 160 lbs. By the time summer had arrived just five or so months later, I was weighing in around 190 to 195 and my strength had gone through the roof in comparison to anything I'd ever felt before (and this was achieved without the use of anabolic steroids). I could reach these gains because I took a true liking to exercise and testing the limitations of the human body. In other words, I executed this challenge by taking on fitness and nutrition as a brand-new way of life.

It was during the first summer home from college when I noticed people didn't always recognize me. It's one thing when you see the progress you've made slowly when looking in the mirror every single day; it's another thing when someone you once knew goes nearly a year without seeing you. I took on a summer job working security at a popular bar/night club in Lake Geneva, Wisconsin, usually covering the front door and checking ID cards on Friday and Saturday nights. Being that I was only 19-years-old, it was hard to imagine a better summer job. Basically, I was paid a modest amount of cash to hang out at a bar, talk to girls, kick out the boyfriends that I didn't like, and listen to trendy music while occasionally sneaking a shot of liquor from the servers. Everything felt like smooth-sailing but it wasn't long until I learned I was rubbing a few folks the wrong way.

My boss at the time called me up one afternoon and bluntly asked me what my deal was. He had numerous, anonymous complaints about me, whether it was drinking too much on the job, non-discreetly letting too many under-age friends through the door, leaving work early to go to some party, etc. It isn't often that in the present moment you fully realize what a cocky loser you can be. I respected my boss, I liked the people I worked with, and I liked many of the customers that came to this place. I was ashamed.

Those wake-up call moments are the ones you may very well end up appreciating later in life because just maybe they were critical in preventing you from getting too carried away. Maybe it was my age, maybe it was the supplements, but most likely it was an ugly combination.

I can't claim that I made all this progress without the help of a few favored supplements. When you're at that young age, the delusional feeling of invincibility overwhelms everything else. I had this willingness to consume almost any over-the-counter supplement that I heard may have had the potential to take me to that next level of achievement. I tried it all; variations of creatine, nitric oxide, testosterone boosters, anything and everything I could get my hands on. I happily tested these products as if I were some laboratory guinea pig, usually without consideration for potential physical/mental harm that could become a serious medical problem later in my life.

It was that same summer home from college that I went to the doctor for my annual physical examination. It was maybe about a week later that I received an alarming telephone call from my physician, explaining that my blood work had returned concerning results; surprise... my liver was inflamed. There was a pause. I asked him if whatever is wrong can be fixed. He replied with something along the lines of; "well, I don't know... you'll have to come in so we can run some more tests".

I remember that feeling like it was yesterday; that tingling sensation you feel in your stomach when you discover you're indeed more vulnerable to danger than you once believed. I also remember agreeing that I would call the doctor back and make an appointment for further examination. I didn't. Right or wrong, I'm the sort of person that will go out of their way to avoid any sort of grim news. On the bright side, immediately after I hung up the phone I promised myself I'd take better care of the delicate life I'd been blessed with.

Of course, being over the age of 18, my parents weren't informed by the office about the current state of my liver and I found no convincing reason to tell them as in my mind all it would do was worry them unnecessarily. I figured the best thing I could do would be to make smarter choices and look out for myself. And you know what? I did; I'm 28 years old and I'm still here and feeling better than ever.

As so many of us know, when we have scary moments like that, it gives us the renewed incentive to appreciate our blessings. I give the "liver episode" credit for being one of the initial triggers that nudged me onto a healthier, and more natural path. I immediately tossed all supplements into the trash and replaced my daily pre-workout supplement with a small cup of pure black coffee. I was shocked to realize that the coffee seemed to have a nearly identical effect and my daily workouts were just as efficient. I was beginning to see a "new light" as it dawned on me that perhaps Rocky Balboa had a valid reason for exercising the old-fashion way, even though many of his rivals were not.

It was with time and consistency that I started to realize that those basic, old-school philosophies for gaining and maintaining lean muscle—which I'll discuss in more detail later—can come with amazing results. It was from this point on that I transitioned my focus to natural fitness and nutrition and I have never looked back. It was because of this newfound focus that I began to despise many of these supplement companies that brainwash so many youngsters into spending exorbitant amounts of money on supplements that, if misused, can have a truly poisonous effect. It also wouldn't surprise me one bit if someone were to discover that half of the unregulated products sold in these supplement stores were nothing more than placebos with attractive packaging.

It wasn't long after I discovered this new passion for fitness that I was frequently approached for advice. It seems most males within that age range (18, 19, 20, etc.) are constantly on the lookout for that 'perfect foolproof formula' that will transform them into looking like some gorilla-juice-head-beefcake. At my current age, I fail to understand why that is, and why I once had the same aspirations. It is obvious why an NCAA athlete, professional athlete or professional body-builder would need that additional size and strength. However, most people in the twenty-first century simply do not require extra mass and in my opinion people who are overly built give off an aura of insecurity.

Friends and acquaintances were consistently questioning me with things like "what do you do for your arms?", "how much cardio do you do?", "how many grams of protein do you consume in one day?". A few close friends would ask me to write them up monthly exercise routines based on their own personal fitness goals. I gave it a shot and to my surprise, I found this quite rewarding and enjoyable. It was always fun for me to see if the plan I created for an individual delivered results (under the proviso that they held themselves accountable and stuck to the regimen).

The downside of this hobby was that it attracted a little too much socialization within the weight room. It got to the point where it seemed that I wasn't ever going to get through my own routine unless I wore a set of headphones, along with a baseball cap tilted downward, covering my eyes. This was an enormous help in hinting to others that I was there to do work. I probably looked like an anti-social psychopath but it was a major aid in terms of helping me to remain focused. Back then, the weight room was therapeutic to me and I wasn't about to lose grasp of that.

It wasn't until my senior year at college that it dawned on me that I could earn a living from something I truly enjoy doing! I still remember the day that I eagerly strolled over to the campus library with a mission to find out what the requirements were for me to become a certified personal trainer. After identifying which institutions in the industry are considered the most prestigious, I checked out every text book I could find, so I could begin to absorb some clinical knowledge. I remember trying to decide what would be more appealing between working as an NFL strength-trainer or opening my own studio-style gym for local, private clients.

There are a wide range of accredited programs out there but in the end, I decided to study for the ACSM (American College of Sports Medicine) certificate since most industry employers throughout the country seemed to not only accept the certificate, but welcome it with open arms.

I had my work cut out for me. I attended seminars, read every affiliated and updated textbook, crammed in countless hours of studying with flash cards and took several practice exams, only to eventually realize that most of the clientele I would be working with were not interested in these specifics. These clients were not looking for someone to regurgitate the scientific mumbo jumbo that I had spent countless hours memorizing; instead, what they wanted was for me to simply show them what to do! They wanted someone to be that person who would hold them accountable for getting to their appointment and breaking a sweat.

In many cases, I'd say the core, prerequisite of your job title as a personal fitness trainer (aside from specialty training categories such as pro-athletes, the mentally-handicapped, etc.) is to be a good listener. I loved that part of the job. I found that you often form a bond with your client when you're consistently bombarded with their worries about their stressful career, the lousy season that their favorite sports team is enduring, or how their husband/wife is constantly nagging. I would often look forward to arriving at work for the social aspect alone.

Shortly after moving to the Big Apple, I applied for a position as a part-time trainer at a rundown, hole-in-the-wall type of gym. Being that I was ACSM certified, I was essentially hired on the spot. This was encouraging as I rapidly took on a solid list of clientele within the first week of employment. The facility was fine; it got the job done and my boss was great, my clients were great, but the less than optimal pay had me feeling like something was missing.

I maybe should have kept my dissatisfaction to myself, as this was only a part-time profession, but the issue was that the gym was charging the clients hefty amounts for 45 minute sessions, and I was only receiving 30 to 40 percent of what these customers were forking over. I continued to bite the bullet. I remember trying to convince myself that I was gaining valuable experience while being paid a little something on the side.

It wasn't long before spring started to bloom. The weather was warming up and NYC residents were looking for any excuse to be outside. A few individual clients began to ask if we could skip the weight room on those nice days and go for a jog or think up some sort of calisthenics (body-weight-exercises) routine that we could perform at the nearby park, which I'm sure went against company policy. They would ask if they could just pay me directly with cash on those days that they preferred to exercise outdoors.

Within the next few months I began to rack in some decent income. Clients that respected my company and work ethic were referring me to friends and associates, and I began to have more and more client inquiries. I was known for being the guy who was flexible with schedules, met you at your home or at the park with resistance bands (which I'll go into detail about later) and charged very modest rates. Departing from that hole-in-the-wall facility was a win-win for myself and my clients; they paid less overall and I profited more overall. I formed very powerful relationships with those clients and I maintain contact with some of them to this day.

It didn't take very long for me to figure out that I thrive best working as an independent contractor; That's just who I am. I prefer to shape my daily schedules without the presence of an employer or supervisor looming over my shoulder. Clearly there are many who prefer that sort of job security, structure, benefits package, etc. and I completely understand that as working for yourself can be intimidating and stressful at times. Even when you manage to get on hot-streaks, you can never be certain how long that success is going to last. That is the price I pay for essentially being able to do whatever I want, whenever I want. We often hear folks make statements about how you're not fully living unless you enjoy what you do for a living; I absolutely stand by that.

As much as I enjoyed working with my client list, my other gig of modeling began to pick up and I became increasingly busy with shoots. New York City is the indisputable mecca of modeling, and models signed with respected agencies are often occupied most days of the week; either going to castings, test-shooting to build their portfolio, or working for catalogs and magazines. At the same time, I was also enrolled in an acting class that held two evening sessions during the week, which made me even less readily available for my fitness clients. Sooner than later I had to choose where my priorities were going to lie. I never truly felt I fit the mold of a "male model". Honestly, I always felt a bit silly posing in front of a camera; it just wasn't me.

The only reason I ever tested those waters was because one of my best buddies from back in Illinois had an older cousin who was earning decent income through an agency in Chicago. Coincidentally, he was also involved in a career as a fitness trainer and took that very seriously. He had opened his own respected training facility in Wisconsin which I had heard was successful. Being able to work in the fitness industry while making some side income through modeling sounded like a great lifestyle to me; It came off as though it would be a "walk in the park". I strolled into a reputable Chicago model agency one day and got lucky; this quickly encouraged me to try my luck in the big market of New York City. Throughout my time working as a model I was lucky enough to shoot for a few well-known companies such as Details

Magazine, Abercrombie & Fitch, Men's Underwear Store, just to name a few.

However, the harsh reality is that very few male models make enough to afford living in New York City. A fair share of men and women model strictly for the opportunity to travel and see the world at a young age. This can be an excellent way to meet people from many other countries as you'll often be living in an agency-leased apartment with bunk beds and three roommates from three different countries. As far as entering the business with the sole intention of making a hefty profit, the odds are stacked heavily against you.

After the economy crashed, many fashion clients that once paid very generous amounts drastically cut their model rates. It seemed that most companies eventually caught on with this strategy which opened the floodgate for industry-wide pay cuts. Models had a choice to either cope with the changing economic climate or leave the industry altogether.

Why would you pay such high rates to a select group of models when there are many other models willing to do the job for free in exchange for some exposure? This became a big industry turn-off for me and many others. I still work a model gig here and there while currently living in Los Angeles, but only through rare direct-bookings as I just can't find the motivation to sit in standstill traffic to attend any more "cattle-call" castings. You walk into any one of those things and it's like hanging out in some sort of depressing hospital waiting room. Everyone (aside from the occasional couple of model "bros" who act like they couldn't be happier to run into each other) is usually completely silent, eyes glued to their smart-phone screens, as they wonder how much more time of their day is going to be wasted before they can hand someone their composite card (the business card of a model). I sure don't miss that part!

On the other hand; not a day goes by that I'm not grateful for being able to dabble in the world of fashion; I made good friends and great connections, experienced NYC living and was ultimately lead to constructing my *nature physique* methods.

Los Angeles, California, had become the "big picture" goal shortly after I enrolled in acting class and so, after two years of living in New York, I made the decision to escape the cold and move out west. I also had the benefit of getting to visit the place on business a few times while

I was living in New York. The warm climate, beach, palm trees and mountains immediately felt right.

To make it even better, two of my hometown pals were looking for a bit of a change as well and immediately jumped on the L.A. bandwagon. The three of us packed our bags, each driving our own car, forming a caravan toward the horizon; it was glorious.

We had agreed to stop in Colorado and camp out for a few nights, which quickly turned into a full week, as I was awestruck by the beautiful and serene environment that surrounded us. We were in our element. It's times like those where you can't help but sit back and reflect on how much there is to be grateful for. It was during this week of being completely immersed in nature that I became truly aware of the sacredness of life and the importance of taking care of your mind, body and soul. Nobody knows how long they have on earth under these beautiful stars. Working your body a little in order to stay physically fit and increase the chance of racking up as many golden memories as possible seems like a no-brainer to me.

Three years have passed since our departure for California. Both of my hometown buddies are currently back in the greater Chicago area, while I remain here in California, living happily with my Australian girlfriend Anna and my two-year old dog- Leeloo. During my time here, I've been lucky enough to work on a few television shows, independent films, and meet some really great people. Hollywood certainly isn't for everyone but I am happy that I have tried out this crazy place while I'm still young.

One specific point that I'd like my readers to walk away with upon finishing this book, is a renewed sense of gratitude not only for their physical fitness and the gift of life but also for the natural world. I'm a firm believer that if most of humanity were to be truly thankful and took the time to regularly get out into nature, this earth would be a much more civilized place.

Gratitude for the blessings in your own life leads to compassion for others. Focus less on what you believe is wrong in your life, and appreciate all things you've been blessed with. This idea is often referred to as the "law of attraction".

Like so many individuals out there, I've experimented with the law of attraction for quite some time now and I am a firm believer. With love, positivity and appreciation as your primary fuel... you can do no wrong.

Upon waking every morning, I simply continue to lie in bed for a couple more minutes. During those few minutes, I create a mental list of all the things both big and small that I'm thankful for. You can list anything from something as minor as the bowl of delicious and nutritious oatmeal that you are about to devour, to as major as the house that you finally managed to finish paying off! You're absolutely guaranteed to get an extra boost which will help get your day off to a positive start!

For an all-around healthy lifestyle... an attitude of gratitude is key.

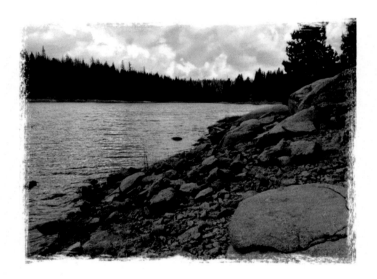

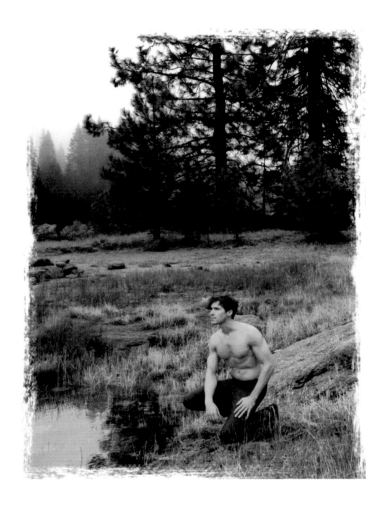

*"Gratitude is not only the greatest of virtues, but
the parent of all others."*

*— Cicero*

Braeden Baade

# Chapter 2 – You Are What You Consume

It's safe to say that the topic of nutrition is one that will be debated forever. With the limitless amount of studies that are released on a daily basis concerning what's deemed "good for you" and what isn't... how are we to really know for certain? One day researchers state that fish oil capsules should be mandatory due to their ability to promote brain health, heart health, etc. As soon as everyone has jumped on that bandwagon, word will spread of a different study stating that fish oil capsules are heavily toxic for the liver, kidneys, and who knows what else? It's this type of constant claim reversal that discourages me (as well as many others) from embracing any trendy, nutritional research as factual. It feels as though one day you're being informed that a

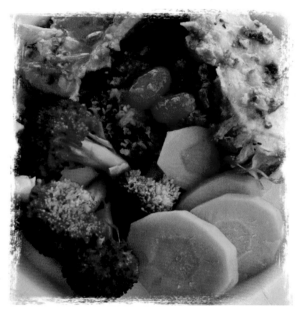

food/vitamin/mineral will block all variations of cancer and you should ABSOLUTELY ingest it three times per day, every day.

Then, before you know it, an entire decade passes, and new studies have discovered that this particular (once almost "miracle-working") nutrient is nothing short of harmful, triggering multiple forms of cancer, and you should toss it into the trash before you breathe any more of the air that it touches! With each year that passes by, the more I find myself shaking my head at the media. I can't even imagine how many dollars are wasted annually because of the silly (and quite possibly harmful) "studies" that flood the public eye.

I want to remind you that by no means am I claiming to know all the science behind nutrition, or that I have a degree to back it up; I don't. What I do want to claim is simply *what has worked for me.*

Back in my earlier days as a meat-headed-psychopath, it was routine for me to consume anything and everything. Whenever I'd visit home during my summers and holidays off from school, I would happily raid the refrigerator and pantry daily. My poor mom was never free from a necessary trip to the grocery store; she practically lived there. That woman is a saint!

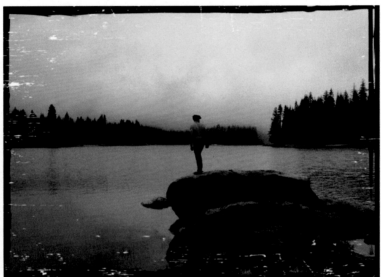

I literally ate whatever meal or snack I could get my hands on and I recall doing it every hour or so as if by clockwork. Now it's important to remember a few things: how young I was, how hard I was conditioning, and even though I ate tons of empty calories... I never neglected the lean and optimal nutrition that is crucial for both gaining and maintaining lean muscle mass; that was always priority number one. Allow me to quickly run you through an example of what I remember my daily intake consisted of. WARNING, this may be disturbing for some!

- **Breakfast:** six raw eggs (I'd gulp them down two at a time), one avocado, one cup of plain steel-cut oatmeal.

- **Morning pre-workout:** cup of black coffee.
- **Post-workout snack:** whey protein shake with at least 20 grams of protein, one banana.
- **Lunch:** broiled chicken breast, 1/2 cup of brown rice, handful of mixed vegetables.
- **Mid-afternoon snack #1:** peanut butter sandwich on whole wheat bread.
- **Mid-afternoon snack #2:** whey protein shake, one apple.
- **Dinner:** Hamburger/steak, corn on the cob, baked potato, handful of mixed vegetables.
- **Before-bed snack:** whey protein shake.
- Wake up... repeat!

You probably just read that and thought to yourself; "wow, that's borderline insane". The best part is this was just the base of what I ate back then; it's what I was referring to as I mentioned "optimal nutrition" above. I snacked on anything and everything in between those base meals to add even more caloric intake.

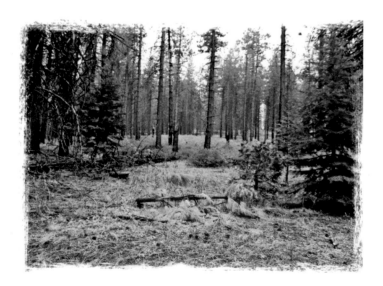

At that time, this meal plan gave me the necessary stamina and strength to match the strenuous resistance training program that I was performing six days out of the week. Due to my naturally-high metabolism, my muscles would've lacked proper recovery without an extreme amount of fuel.

It would probably be appropriate now to give you a sigh of relief; the *nature physique* meal plan example that I've listed is nothing like that! After-all, if you're reading this book, your goal is most certainly not to transform into an enormous, ape-like beast. Rest assured that this next layout will illustrate what I currently consume throughout my day to reach and maintain a slim, but solid *nature physique*.

Again, it's important to remember that I'm not claiming to be a dietitian or nutritionist; This is purely what has worked for ME from my own experience. Choose to mimic at your own risk, and of course be mindful of any food allergies you may have.

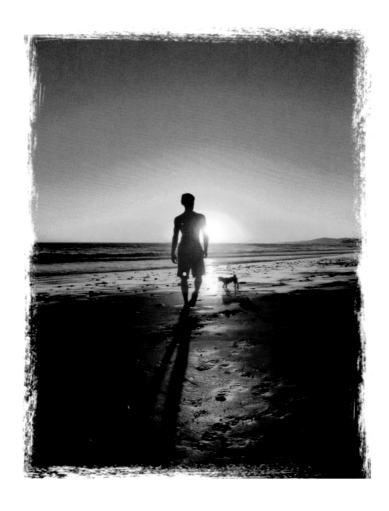

# *Nature Physique* Meal Plan Example

- **Breakfast:** one cup of plain Greek yogurt, mixed with a handful of blueberries, and one tablespoon of chia seeds.
- **Morning pre-workout:** one cup of black coffee, or one cup of green tea.
- **Post-workout snack:** whey protein shake containing at least 20 grams of protein.
- **Lunch:** choose between a grilled/broiled chicken breast, salmon fillet, pork chop, handful of steamed vegetables or salad, and 1/2 avocado.
- **Mid-afternoon snack:** one apple with one spoonful of peanut butter, or a pouch of unsalted almonds.
- **Dinner:** choose between filet mignon, grilled/broiled salmon, grilled/broiled chicken breast, or pork chop, spinach salad with a light balsamic vinaigrette dressing, and a handful of steamed vegetables.

From my experience, this is an excellent meal plan that keeps my metabolism high, energy levels up, and helps to suppress the craving of sweets and other junk foods. You don't need to replicate it every single day, but the point is to display an example that you can use as a base to mix and match with; just try to use common sense on what would be healthy options like the items listed above. The big picture goal here is to, over time, convince your body that you're consuming enough nutritious calories on a regular basis, thus relieving it from thinking it constantly needs to hold on to excess calories for survival purposes. The human body's main concern is not to show off prominent core muscles or biceps; the human body's only true objective is to *survive.*

Another useful tip to help satisfy unnecessary cravings is to make sure you're receiving adequate water throughout the day. Staying hydrated goes a long way in terms of helping you feel full.

# For Vegetarians

Because I've listed a good amount of meat within the previous meal plans, I thought it would be fair to create one for vegetarians. I have been known to go through vegetarian cycles myself that I estimate last between three weeks and a month per phase. I usually do this as a method of detoxifying or "shocking" my body; whether it has any physical benefit, or is just strictly mental... I'm not completely sure. But I do feel good by switching it up occasionally.

Obviously, the tricky part of a vegetarian diet is ensuring that you are consuming enough protein to fully recover from your exercise routine. If you don't consistently receive a good amount, strenuous exercise tends to backfire on the body. When on a vegetarian diet, I make sure to have access to plenty of protein-rich foods like quinoa, peanut butter, tree nuts, chick peas, a variety of beans, etc.

Below is an example of a meal plan that I find to be satisfactory when on a vegetarian routine. You'll notice it's quite like the previous meal plan with the only primary difference being that you're substituting the meat with a vegetarian alternative.

- **Breakfast:** choose between ½ cup of steel-cut oatmeal or one cup of plain Greek yogurt, with ½ cup of fresh berries, and one tablespoon of chia seeds.
- **Morning pre-workout:** one cup of black coffee or, one cup of green tea.
- **Post-workout snack:** whey protein shake with at least 20 grams of protein, and one banana or one apple.
- **Lunch:** one bowl of quinoa, mixed with chopped sweet potato, mushrooms, and spinach.
- **Mid-afternoon snack:** one apple, with one tablespoon of peanut butter or almond butter.
- **Dinner:** black bean salad, mixed with avocado, corn, cherry tomatoes, bell pepper, red onion, and cilantro leaves.

# Gluten Free

Since the idea of being gluten-free has become so trendy within the last decade or so, I thought it would be groovy to include an example of what a gluten-free *nature physique* meal plan could look like.

I will say I've gone through cycles of experimenting on the exclusion of gluten and I am not too certain I ever found it to have any noticeable impact, physically or mentally. That's not to say that there aren't plenty of people out there that have found it to be beneficial within some aspect of every-day-living. Of course, gluten allergies do exist and those always need to be taken into careful consideration, therefore it seemed worthy to discuss a routine targeted toward those "GF" folks!

However, here is a nice little surprise; the previous two meal plans are indeed gluten-free. So if you're a happy "GF" individual, you won't feel like you're missing out at all. It's been to my experience that if you tend to avoid most processed foods in general, you're automatically going to avoid a large fraction of items containing gluten. Because of this, I'd say I'm unintentionally gluten-free most days of the week.

# Easy on the Salt

Another topic that I've found important enough to mention is that of sodium intake. Health-wise, it's widely known that excess sodium can increase risk of undesirable consequences such as; headaches, kidney stones, stroke, osteoporosis, heart disease, and others. Appearance-wise, it can trigger weight gain, bloating, and puffiness. In America, it seems to be a cultural norm to add an abundance of salt to our dish. Inconveniently enough, this is a dilemma we need to constantly take into consideration because it can be tricky to avoid. If you do certain things on the regular like consume fast food, packaged food, or eat at sit-down restaurants... chances are that your sodium intake is through the roof.

There is a common belief that if we limit our sodium intake to under 2300 mg per day (or 1500 mg if age 51 or over), we can greatly decrease the risk of the unwanted effects. The obstacle with this is that it's very challenging to remain under these sodium levels if we dine out at a restaurant even once per day. Now, if you insist on adding salt to every meal and can't possibly imagine that anything will taste up to par without it, I'm not implying that the work you've put into obtaining your *nature physique* is completely pointless; all I'm saying is that maybe in some cases a little moderation could go a long way.

Home cooking is almost always your best bet, as you can obviously monitor exactly what goes into each meal. If you use a variety of spices, you may very well discover there is little to no need for added salt, and over time, you're taste buds will begin to adjust and even thank you!

As Americans, many of us go through life (at least during the earlier years) completely ignorant to the overwhelming amount of sodium which we absorb day in and day out. It isn't until we act to exclude it that we begin to see the benefits. As for myself, I grew up on an extremely high sodium diet. My parents, and grandparents (whom I visited nearly every single weekend) were so busy with work most of the time that we often had no alternative but to either eat out at a restaurant or throw some prepackaged meal into the oven or microwave. Some of my most vivid childhood memories are of my grandfather picking me up after school on Friday afternoons and taking me to McDonald's to get an order of fries. When you think of McDonald's fries, one of the first ingredients that most likely comes to mind is salt. The funny thing is that I remember my grandpa would pour the fries into a bag, then empty not one, but TWO packets of salt into the bag and shake it all up until the fries were smothered in even more sodium! I used to absolutely love this; it was almost addictive and tasted so good back then. It wasn't until later in life, when I took initiative to making healthier choices, that I began to get word of the negative effects of excess sodium.

Not only did I ditch the addition of salt, but I began to review every single nutrition label (the ones I could get my hands on) of the food items I consumed. To not much surprise, I found the results were almost instantaneous; overall more hydrated, my body wasn't as puffy, and my mouth no longer felt like the Sahara Desert. As I'm sure you've noticed on many occasions, the inside of the mouth tends to dry up after meals that are heavy in salt.

Take note that the more water you drink, the more easily your body can flush out unwanted sodium.

# Alcohol: Good or Evil?

It's safe to say that when someone dives into a new fitness routine, they often wonder if alcohol consumption is still an option. That's completely up to you. As with most things, I strongly believe that moderation is another key element here. I do drink alcohol here and there. Whether it's having a beer or two while watching football, or having a glass or two of red wine when out to dinner, I'll usually indulge. But I do know my limits and that is something you always need to consider for yourself.

Some claim that it's not actually the alcohol itself that encourages the weight-gain, but rather the unhealthy, sodium-rich, greasy or perhaps fried foods that are often consumed in unison with alcohol intake. This is because, upon ingestion, the human body simply recognizes all forms of alcohol as poison. For example, say you're currently plowing through a tray of buffalo wings during the big game. During this consumption, or slightly after, you decide to wash all that spice down with a few beers. Your liver will immediately remove full focus from the digestion of the wings and instead focus on metabolizing the alcohol to flush it out of your system.

The liver is unable to efficiently metabolize fat while occupied with metabolizing alcohol. The issue with this interruption of the liver is that it often leads to the food calories being ignored, set aside, and stored unnecessarily within the tissue. It's one of the main contributors to why we commonly come across what is referred to as a 'skinny-fat' person. A 'skinny-fat' person is someone whom appears extremely thin with a shirt on (thin arms, neck, shoulders, legs, etc.), but when the shirt is removed, we often notice the form of a 'beer-belly' (a stomach that appears to protrude in comparison to the rest of the body).

Clearly there are many alcoholic beverages out there that are more or less unhealthy than others. Personally (and I'm definitely not alone here), if I'm going to have a few drinks, I tend to stay away from anything with a high sugar content. Sugary drinks tend to give me a headache and it feels as if my body has more difficulty flushing it out. Luckily they don't taste very appealing to me either! I'll almost always stick to a nice ale or lager.

I might sound crazy for saying this, but sometimes I feel as though I have an even better workout the following day if I drank a couple beers (literally just a COUPLE) the previous night. To help rid you of some guilt for consuming the occasional couple of beers, I have added a list of some of the many beer-drinking-benefits:

- **High in fiber:** Not only is a moderate amount of beer good for your digestive health, but it also works as an appetite suppressant. This will aid in helping the body feel fuller for longer periods, thus preventing over-eating. Further, this type of fiber is believed to lower cholesterol, while also improving overall heart health. For even more fiber, go for darker beer!
- **Reduces risk of type-2 diabetes:** Rumor has it that moderate beer-drinkers lower their risk of acquiring type-2 diabetes by a whopping 30%.
- **Increases bone density:** Some claim that, due to the hefty silicon content, moderate beer drinkers have a better chance of building and maintaining stronger bones in comparison to those who don't drink beer at all. Because of this, it is believed that beer may contribute to the fight against osteoporosis. Again, there is a large emphasis on **MODERATION** and I can't stress that enough. This needs to be clear due to fact that the same studies discovered that frequent, excess beer consumption can backfire and lead to the weakening of the bones
- **Reduces stress:** This benefit is more to do with moderate alcohol consumption in general rather than particularly to beer. About 24 ounces of alcohol per day for men, and about 12 ounces per day for women, can commonly lead to minimization of stress and/or anxiety.

I want to be clear that I'm not advocating for beer to be placed at the top of the food pyramid, nor am I stating that you will reap every possible benefit without any possible side effects. Of course, we all know that frequent alcohol consumption is harmful to the liver. All I ask is that you feel at ease after cracking open the occasional beer or two while on a fitness regimen; your path toward your *nature physique* shall not suffer.

# Cheat Meal Days

Another popular topic of discussion for my fitness clients was that of the infamous "cheat meal" or "cheat day". If you're not familiar with this expression, it involves the theory that you should allow yourself the pleasure of eating one meal out of the week that is calorie-dense and is also something you deeply desire. This meal is meant to serve not only as a reward for having remained disciplined during the rest of the week, but also to "shock" your metabolism when you feel as though you've reached a plateau in your fitness progress. Whatever the goal is that you're working toward, this plateau can culminate in the of lack of further weight-loss, lack of further strength increase or lack of further muscle mass increase. A cheat meal can often be an effective aid if you begin to feel the symptoms of overtraining.

Overtraining symptoms can easily occur if the body feels as though it's lacking in the nutrients that are needed to recover from consistent exercise. These symptoms include insomnia, irritability, depression, physical injury, etc. It would be practical to assume that a cheat meal would be totally counterproductive on a weight-loss or shredding regimen but it can encourage your body to keep reaching for new heights. I do this all the time. When asked what my go-to cheat meal after a productive week would commonly be I almost always answer with "Chipotle burrito... extra guacamole". Aside from the taste, the calorie amount is so substantial that I just can't help but feel physically-satisfied and revitalized for yet another productive week.

The best aspect of implementing a cheat meal is that you don't have to feel guilty for stuffing yourself since your metabolism will be more conditioned, due to the frequent intake of nutritious calories.

It has been to my perception that you are at the greatest risk for hitting an over-training plateau if you are on a weight-loss routine and are not mindful of moderation. If you're not careful, it can be extremely easy to get carried away and deprive your body of the nutrition it needs to sustain healthy progress.

# Green Tea: My Pre-Workout Beverage

Once you've made consistent exercise a life necessity, you may discover that you've acquired certain pre-workout rituals. My ritual is that I must always drink green tea within the 30 minutes before beginning my workout. The dense antioxidant and caffeine combination supplies my body with the fuel to help me stay focused and energized throughout my workout. Even aside from exercise, I tend to sip on green tea throughout my day to reap the many health benefits. Truth be told; I'm currently sipping on a fresh cup as I write this sentence.

Green tea is known as one of the oldest forms of natural, herbal medicine. It is praised for its countless health benefits and is extremely popular among Asian and American cultures. Although black tea consistently remains the most popular tea beverage within the United States, green tea reigns supreme for having the highest concentration of powerful antioxidants. This is partially due to the fermentation process that black tea must go through before it becomes available to consumers. Since green tea doesn't need to be fermented, it can hold onto much of its antioxidants.

Although not all the proceeding green tea health benefits can yet be deemed as 100% factual, there is substantial evidence to indicate that they are indeed a reality. As an avid green tea consumer of many years, I can vouch that the wonderful, green substance does nothing but good for my body and mind.

# Green Tea Benefits

## *Encourages healthy brain function*

Like coffee, the primary ingredient in green tea is caffeine. Although it normally contains less caffeine than coffee, many folks find it to be a desirable alternative in the sense that it still allows for improved focus and energy while excluding certain undesirable effects such as "the jitters". From what I can tell, a healthy dosage of caffeine can lead to advancements in memory, mood, and reaction time. Green tea also includes a valuable amino acid known as L-theanine which is claimed to be responsible for helping to reduce feelings of anxiety while increasing the levels of dopamine (a chemical found in the brain that triggers positive feelings). Together, caffeine and L-theanine form a wonderful partnership, working cooperatively to improve overall brain activity, thus making green tea a particularly ideal beverage. Interestingly, many consumers claim that they feel a sense of stability in their energy levels and productivity when they select green tea over coffee. I couldn't agree more!

## Could decrease risk of cardiovascular disease

Some folks suggest that daily green tea consumption may help to encourage a healthy balance of cholesterol within the body. This is due to improvement in overall blood-flow, as well as an improved antioxidant release within the blood. By acquiring good cholesterol, risk of heart disease is substantially diminished.

## May lead to fat loss

If you were to do some research on what common products aid in the elimination of body fat, the chances are good that you would come across multiple recommendations for green tea. This is largely due to green tea increasing metabolic activity. The potent combination of antioxidants and caffeine trigger the beneficial response of activating fatty acids that have been stored within the bodily tissues. Fat is actually a very valuable source of energy but is not always efficiently converted into energy. If the human body can effectively convert fat into energy on a regular basis, fat loss will naturally follow. Not a bad side effect if you ask me!

## Rids the body of harmful bacteria

Let's face it; bacteria is everywhere. I do everything I can to maintain a healthy defense against the intrusion of harmful bacteria. This involves thoroughly and constantly washing my hands, consuming a daily multi-vitamin, eating nutritious foods, getting adequate sleep, etc. Green tea is believed to act as another shield when fighting off pesky germs. For example; one of the most common places for unwanted bacteria to settle is inside the mouth. This type is known as streptococcus mutans and is guilty of triggering plaque buildup. As we all know, plaque is often to blame for annoying consequences such as tooth decay and cavities. Studies indicate that green tea is effective in preventing the growth of this specific bacteria, keeping teeth and gums clean and furthermore eliminating cases of bad breath! In some cases, green tea is also believed to greatly lower the risk of intrusive viruses, as well as prevent infection.

## Fights against allergies

Green tea is believed to be an effective warrior when it comes to limiting the effects of stubborn allergies. This belief is primarily credited to a compound called epigallocatechin gallate (or abbreviated as EGCG). It is said to be most effective against common allergic reactions such as those triggered by pollen.

## Enhances eyesight

Turns out that carrots aren't the only dietary substance that can improve our vision. The potent antioxidant known as catechins, may indeed contribute to eye health. This may take place due to the eye's ability to absorb catechins into its tissue.

## Protects against harmful UV rays

In addition to sunscreen, green tea is said to work as an extra guard when warding off UV radiation. The catechins that are found in green tea can form an added resistance for the skin and potentially reduce the effects from skin aging. Make sure you don't forget your iced green tea beverage during your next visit to the beach!

Now don't get me wrong; I know plenty of people that will almost always choose coffee as their pre-workout beverage, and they do just fine with that. Coffee has been claimed to have a boatload of health benefits and is able to help you stay focused during your exercise routine. I've experimented with green tea and coffee many, many times up to this point and simply feel as though my body reacts more advantageously to green tea. I enjoy the stability in terms of the energy I receive from the tea. For me, coffee delivers too much stimulation all at once, thus leading me to a lethargic state within the coming hours. Obviously, a more intense caffeine rush is appealing to many. Everyone has a preference; it's important to find out what works best for you.

If you are a consistent coffee drinker and can't see yourself performing some trial and error with the alternative green tea anytime soon, I would absolutely recommend that you at least try consuming coffee in its purest form (black) without any added dairy or added sweeteners. This will not only cut out excess (and pointless) calories, but it will allow for quicker and less diluted absorption of the desired content such as caffeine and antioxidants, thus potentially triggering a more productive training session. It can also help to drastically reduce the chance of stomach cramps while performing an exercise routine.

Whether you're a green tea or coffee person, you may want to consider that there is said to be a list of potential health risks when consuming daily amounts of excess caffeine. A general rule of thumb for recommended daily caffeine dosage is to remain within 200 to 300 milligrams; this is equivalent to roughly three to four cups of coffee. When someone constantly consumes more than this recommended amount, they're vulnerable to a spectrum of unwanted side effects such as irritability, rapid heart rate, and trouble with sleeping.

Like I stated before, I manage better when I stay green!

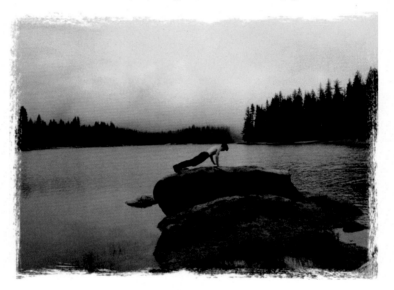

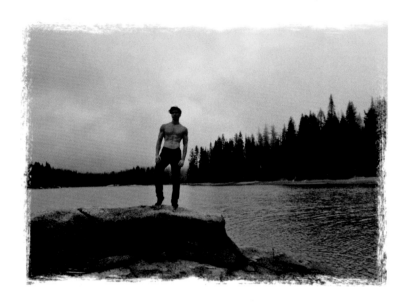

*"You need to listen to your body because your body is listening to you."*

*— Phillip C. McGraw*

Braeden Baade

# Chapter 3 – Which Body Type Are You?

When you take the time to stroll through an urban area, you will absolutely notice a wide range of shapes and sizes when it comes to the human physique. But things would get a whole lot more interesting if you could somehow visualize how everyone would appear if they were to completely exclude exercise and nutritious choices from their daily lives.

Since way back in time, there are said to be three different human body types. This theory includes that of the ectomorph, endomorph, and mesomorph. An ectomorph is generally very 'thin', an endomorph is generally on the 'rounder' side, and a mesomorph is generally on the 'bulkier' or naturally-muscular side of the spectrum. Which one are you? Well it's important to remember that most of us don't all fall entirely into one specific type. In fact we can commonly carry particular traits from each. However, most us tend to fall somewhere in between two out of the three forms.

It is believed that in order to figure out your body's type, you must think back to the build that you possessed while you were in your adolescence; the physique that you naturally represented well before diet, exercise, and aging effects all played major parts in the shape that you acquired so many years later. For example, I believe myself to originally fall into the ectomorphic classification. As a child, I was extremely scrawny; I'd eat anything and everything and fail to put on any added muscle mass, or added weight for that matter. But when I applied basic exercise and nutrition principles in my late teenage years, I noticed that I had a multitude of mesomorph traits hidden within. Upon consuming the nutritious and necessary protein-rich foods, while incorporating a resistance training regimen, my body responded in a way where it almost seemed as if it had been waiting a long time to become something it had never been before.

It can be somewhat important to understand what body type you represent to properly evaluate the type of routine that will be most beneficial for you. However, I want to make it clear that I believe all forms of exercise to be beneficial if you remain careful to prioritize safety and consistently avoid over-training. There is always a safe and effective way to train.

The following pages consist of information on the three general body types, including specific traits, as well as pictures to help you in determining your category.

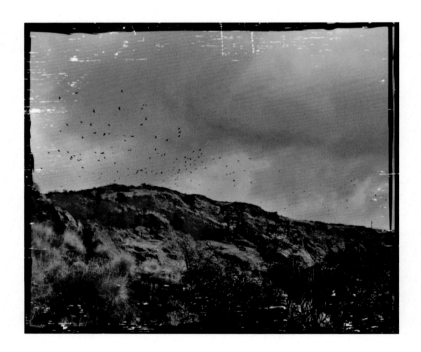

# The Ectomorph

Appearance:

- Extremely low body fat.
- Narrower face.
- Heightened forehead.
- Thin chest and core.
- Legs are often longer in relation to the torso.
- Narrower shoulders

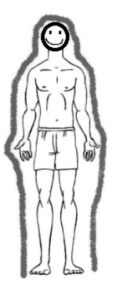

Exercise for the ectomorph:

- Exhaust each muscle no more than once per week (the ectomorphic build generally requires longer recovery periods in comparison to the others). However, I would exclude abdominal and core muscles from this notion as I find that they can and should be worked more often (at least from my experience).
- It's extremely important to hold off on training a muscle if the designated muscle is sore from a recent workout.
- Alter the exercise routine monthly.
- Keep extreme cardiovascular exercise to a minimum, as it can be counteractive for the ectomorph in terms of building muscle. The ectomorph metabolism is often very productive when it comes to burning calories; therefore, it's advantageous to limit the amount of nutritious calories (used for muscle building) that escape the body.

# The Endomorph

Appearance:

- Wide frame/bone structure.
- Wider hips.
- Narrower shoulders.
- Many fatty areas, hiding the muscle beneath.

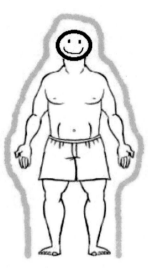

Exercise for the endomorph:

- It's important for the endomorph to train quite frequently as this will help to counteract against this body types' slower metabolism. Due to the endomorph's tendency to store fat, consistent cardiovascular exercise is highly beneficial.
- The endomorph responds well to higher intensity. This translates to shorter rest periods between sets.
- Resistance training and aerobic training routines can be altered on a constant basis as it's important for the endomorph's muscles to be regularly "shocked".
- Full body workouts are appealing to the endomorphic build in the sense that they almost always trigger a heightened heart rate.
- An endomorph should always work the abdominal and core muscles at the beginning of a routine; this tactic will help to ensure that they're done effectively and/or not neglected.

# The Mesomorph

Appearance:

- Naturally muscular build.
- Larger head.
- Narrower waist.
- Broader shoulders.
- Minimal body fat.
- Solid chest.

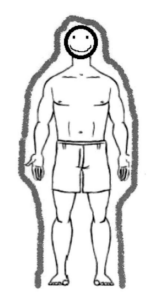

Exercise for the mesomorph:

- For the mesomorph, most muscle groups respond extremely well to keeping the repetitions count to 12 or under.
- It's highly beneficial for this build to incorporate a wide variety of exercises. The more, the better, as the mesomorph is believed to be able to stay in an anabolic state for longer periods of time than the other body types.
- If looking to add muscle, it's important for this body type to not overdo it when it comes to aerobic training. Like the ectomorph body type, the mesomorph can plateau if too many calories are burned during intense cardiovascular activity. It could be beneficial to limit aerobic training to about three sessions in a week.

Braeden Baade

# Chapter 4 – Warming Up and Dynamic Stretching

Before I get into my favorite resistance training routines, it's crucial that I don't neglect the importance of warming up with dynamic stretching, followed by a quick cardiovascular exercise. By making this a tradition, you will be allowing your body to carefully transition into an anabolic state (also known as the muscle-building state), thus encouraging optimum blood-flow, lubrication of the joints, and more elasticity within the muscles. In other words, you will always have a more productive resistance training session after setting aside the time to warm up. It will also help to prevent pulled muscles and other injuries.

Upon completing my dynamic stretch, I like to proceed with either a light five to ten-minute jog/jump rope session, or if I don't have adequate space, 100 jumping jacks. The key is to increase your heart rate just enough to build a sweat to lubricate the muscles and joints, as well as improve overall blood-flow.

The following page contains photos of my preferred dynamic stretches. Feel free to mix and match to create an order that is to your liking.

# Dynamic Stretching
Make sure to perform these stretches with a smooth and careful motion.

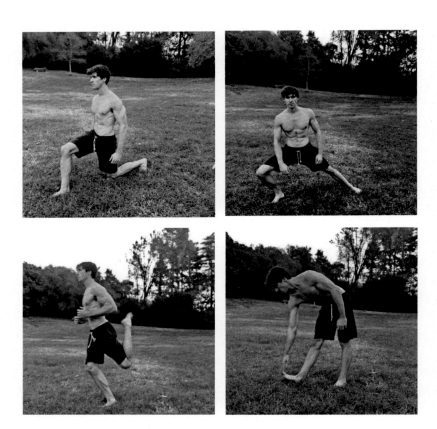

# Chapter 5 – Sculpting your Nature Physique

Now for the juicy part, and most likely primary reason as to why you're reading this book in the first place; the exercise routines. Be assured that you don't need any fancy equipment to execute these exercises with full precision. What you do need is a patch of grass, a beautiful, sturdy tree, a set of resistance bands, and finally; commitment.

Sculpting your body into its *nature physique* is not meant to be perceived as a chore; it is meant to be savored as both a therapeutic and enjoyable part of your day. It's important that you always embrace the sweat, buildup of lactic acid, and increase in heart rate as positive changes taking place within the body. If you can persistently harness this mentality, you will find it much easier to stay motivated.

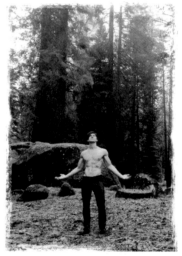

The proceeding sections are comprised of a variety of training routines. Dive into whichever looks appealing and comfortable to you. Whatever routine you choose to take on first, I recommend you switch to a different routine every four to six weeks. By doing so, you will be encouraging your muscles to adapt to new challenges, thus continuing on the path of progress.

My hope is that, after time, you will no longer need to refer to these pages, as these exercises will find a way of imprinting within your mind. You may even discover that, as time passes, your creativity will kick in and you'll obtain enough experience points to construct your own customized routines! That is totally cool, and I absolutely condone it!

# *Nature Physique* Interval Training

Interval training is typically performed by combining a series of anaerobic exercises (an exercise intense enough to trigger lactic acid buildup). The goal behind interval training is to incorporate an increase in muscular strength, while simultaneously increasing cardiovascular endurance. In my opinion, it is a suitable program for someone whom is looking to build muscle, maintain a healthy heart, cut calories, and find a way of doing so in a timely manner.

When constructing these interval training routines, I made it a point to incorporate the core muscles (abs, obliques, etc.) within each one. For so many, the idea of acquiring prominent abdominal muscles is a heavily sought-after desire and was one of the most frequent topics during fitness consultation when I spent my earlier days as a personal trainer.

Because these interval routines exhaust multiple muscle groups, I'd recommend engaging in these workouts no more than three days out of the week. For example; you could choose to perform them Monday, Wednesday, Friday... then repeat the following week. Many of my clients preferred a three day per week program and never failed to see encouraging progress.

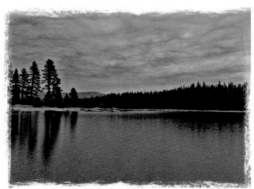

If your primary goal is to lose weight and/or shred your core, I'd recommend implementing simple cardiovascular exercise during your "off-days". For example, you could go for a light, 30-minute bicycle ride, improve your agility and endurance with the use of a jump-rope, or even participate in a basketball game or tennis match with friends. Finding the time to consistently "break a sweat" six to seven days out of the week will work wonders for your physique, your mind, and all-around sense of well-being.

# The *Nature Physique* Interval Routines

The *nature physique* interval routine is crafted toward beginners and/or individuals who are looking to perform a light resistance routine combined with mild cardiovascular output. As your muscles begin to adapt to this routine, you'll want to implement some alterations such as an increase in the number of repetitions, time spent in plank position, amount of sets using the heavier bands, and even the order of exercises. Listen to your body and you will know when the alterations are necessary. If the circuit starts to become too easy, that's a good sign that your muscles are developing and it's time to switch it up.

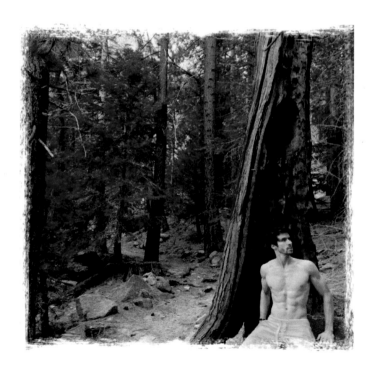

# Interval Circuit #1 (Monday)

Interval circuit #1 primarily targets the quadriceps, pectorals, glutes, deltoids, and core. I would recommend getting into a habit of performing this circuit on Mondays. That way it is easy to remember to do interval circuit #2 on Wednesday, followed by interval circuit #3 on Friday.

This circuit includes the following exercises:
1) Tree stump lunge - 30 reps
2) Resistance band chest press - 30 reps
3) Prisoner squats - 30 reps
4) Resistance band upright row - 30 reps
5) Plank - hold for 30 seconds
— Rest for 60 seconds, then repeat the circuit.

- Have a stopwatch on hand (a smart phone works quite well).
- Repeat the circuit three times.
- Perform the first cycle with the lightest resistance band, second cycle with the middleweight band, and third cycle with heavyweight band.

# Exercise #1: Tree Stump Lunge

In this *nature physique* twist on the traditional lunge, I prefer to use a tree stump as a general guide; an object to reach for while performing the exercise. Clearly, this can be done just as effectively with a cone or any other object that is comparable in height. The point of the object is to help ensure that you are getting low enough to the ground to increase the muscles' range of motion.

- Begin by locating a flat surface and make sure your feet are hip-width apart.
- relax your shoulders and back, stand straight, engage your core and encourage good posture.
- Place one hand on top of the other, fingers together and pointing outward (creating an arrow shape). Raise them straight above your head as seen in the photo.
- Start the motion by stepping forward with your right foot to a distance that will allow for your left knee to almost touch the ground. At the same time, lower your locked hands downward as if you were almost reaching for the tree stump in front of you. Now, in one fluid motion return to the starting position of standing up straight with hands in the arrow position, above your head, pointed toward the sky.
- Repeat with left foot.

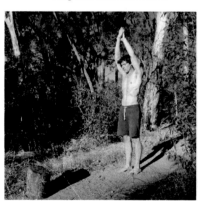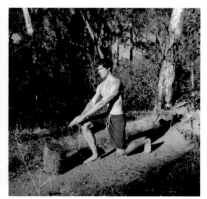

# Exercise #2: Resistance Band Chest Press

This exercise is a great alternative to the basic push up. It targets the same muscle groups (pectorals, shoulders, and triceps) but allows for better support as gravity isn't working against you. As much as I love pushups, they can sometimes be strenuous on the shoulders and if you're relatively new to resistance training, chances are you'll be able to perform the resistance band chest press with better form. Once you become an expert with the resistance band chest press and have developed the targeted muscles, you may want to consider substituting this exercise with basic pushups as a strategy to further shock the body and overcome any plateaus.

- Begin by locating a firm, stationary base to wrap the resistance band around. A sturdy tree with a narrower girth will work in your favor. If you don't have a tree available to you, or you need to exercise indoors there are a wide range of substitutes that can be used in place of a tree.
- Face your back toward the tree, place one foot out in front of the other to encourage a balanced stance, and grip the handles in a way that allows for the band to be positioned under your forearms and elbows.
- Raise your elbows to the point of creating a 90-degree angle between your arms and your body.
- Start the motion by pushing the grips forward until your arms have straightened outward in front of you.
- Reverse the motion by allowing the bands to retract inward back toward the body.

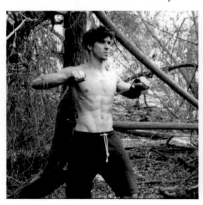 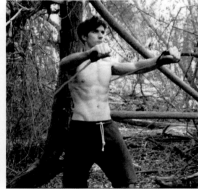

# Exercise #3: Prisoner Squats

This exercise is an incredibly convenient and effective one in the sense that it's safe, works a multitude of muscles, and can be done literally anywhere. I consider it to be one of the best exercises for working the quadriceps, glutes, hamstrings, and core.

- Locate a flat surface.
- Begin by getting into a shoulder-width stance with your toes directed slightly outward.
- Position your hands behind your head (as if you were being held up by a police officer) and gently hold them there throughout the duration of the exercise.
- Keep your torso in an upright position while allowing for a slight arch in the lower back, as you'll want your butt to be pointing outward during the motion.
- Initiate the motion by carefully bending your legs downward until the hips fall just below the knee level. Then, in a powerful but careful motion, explode upward to the starting position.
- Repeat.

NOTE: During this exercise, it is important to remember to position your weight onto your heels. Take extra special care to ensure that your heels never leave the ground throughout the motion.

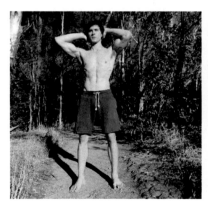 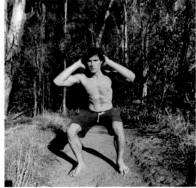

# Exercise #4: Resistance Band Upright Row

This exercise specifically targets the top portion of the deltoids (shoulders) and increases muscular endurance for the 'pulling' motion. I wanted to make sure to incorporate an exercise where the shoulder muscles are isolated since they're already being worked during this circuit.

- Begin by locating a flat surface.
- Form a stance that is shoulder-width apart. Place the middle of the resistance band carefully under your feet (I recommend wearing shoes for this exercise as it can be somewhat uncomfortable for bare feet). Make sure the band's tension feels balanced on both sides of your body.
- While maintaining good posture, raise your hands until they nearly meet your collarbone. For optimal form, attempt to consistently raise the elbows slightly higher than the hands. This will trigger more of the muscle's range of motion.
- Gently lower your arms all the way down to the starting point before carefully exploding back upward.
- Repeat.

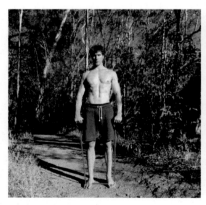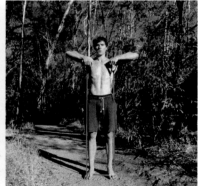

# Exercise #5: Plank

This basic but incredibly effective exercise is heavily praised for the wonders it does to the core. Not only is it one of the most efficient ways to obtain a prominent six-pack, it strengthens the entire body; especially the lower back and shoulders. Many folks find planks to be rather grueling but well worth it when they discover the relatively quick results. As with many other exercises, it becomes noticeably easier over time. Make sure to have some sort of stopwatch next to you so that you can focus your mind elsewhere as opposed to relying on yourself to accurately count down the seconds.

- Begin by locating a flat but comfortable surface. A spot on the grass, carpet, or yoga mat should work perfectly.
- Create a 90-degree bend in your elbows and focus your weight onto your forearms.
- Make sure that your body forms a straight line all the way from your neck to your feet.
- An excellent way to further verify correct form can be done by lining up your elbows to where they are positioned directly below your shoulders.
- Initiate the pose by lifting your knees from the ground, holding this position for 30 seconds. If you find the 30 second period to be too easy for you, great; go for 60 seconds. With time and practice, the goal should be to eventually gain the ability to hold the plank pose for two minutes. Coming from my experience, you'll be pleasantly surprised at how fast this exercise strengthens your core.

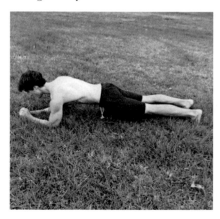

# Interval Circuit #2 (Wednesday)

Interval circuit #2 targets the muscles of the back, biceps, calves, and core. It is meant to be performed no sooner than 48 hours after completing interval circuit #1. This will allow for the body to have had adequate recovery time before exhausting the following muscle groups.

This circuit includes the following exercises:
1) Resistance band lat pulldown - 30 reps
2) Resistance band woodchopper - 30 reps on each side (for a total of 60 reps)
3) Resistance band standing bicep curl - 30 reps
4) Standing calf raise - 50 reps
5) Basic crunch - 30 reps
— Rest for 60 seconds, then repeat the circuit.

- Have a stopwatch on hand (a smart phone works quite well).
- Repeat the circuit three times.
- Perform the first cycle with the lightest resistance band, second cycle with the middleweight band, and third cycle with the heavyweight band.

# *Exercise #1: Resistance Band Lat Pulldown*

This exercise is an easier variation of the basic pull-up as it works the muscles of the upper back. Once you are accustomed to this workout and feel as though you've strengthened the targeted muscles, you may want to consider substituting this exercise with the basic pull-up. This will help to further shock the muscles and potentially reach new gains.

- Begin by locating a sturdy tree branch that is within reaching distance, as you'll need to loop the resistance band a couple feet above your head (remember that the higher the branch, the stronger the resistance). The branch can also be lower than head level if you'd like to perform the exercise while in a kneeling position.
- Grasp the handles and position your hands so that they are a bit wider than shoulder-width.
- Initiate the motion by pulling down the handles until your elbows nearly contact your torso.
- Gently allow the resistance to pull the band all the way back upward to the starting position.
- Repeat.

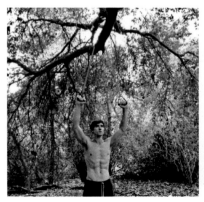 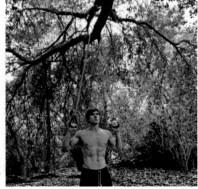

# Exercise #2: Resistance Band Woodchopper

This exercise is an excellent one for improving core strength and toning the oblique muscles (the muscles that run alongside the abdomen). Since the abdominal muscles usually attract far more attention, I thought it would be beneficial to incorporate an exercise that targets the body's 'twisting' range of motion. It's important to work all those little foundation muscles just as hard to maintain proportion and balance.

- Begin by locating a sturdy tree; wrap the band around the tree and loop one handle through the other to create a secure anchor. If you don't have a tree available, place one end of the band in between a door and the door frame (make sure the door is tightly closed).
- Position your body so that your right side is facing the tree (or door), spread your feet shoulder-width apart.
- To begin the motion, grasp the resistance band handle with both hands and smoothly swing it across your body, mimicking the motion of swinging an axe. Remember to maintain a loose posture by gently bending the knees and twisting throughout the waist.
- Gently return to the starting position.
- Repeat with the opposite side.

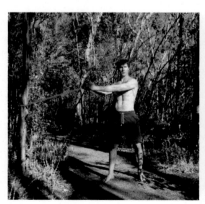
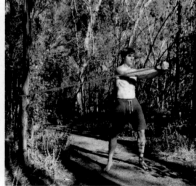

# Exercise #3: Resistance Band Standing Bicep Curl

This basic exercise is one of my favorites as it primarily targets the biceps and forearms. It's another incredibly convenient exercise as it can be done anywhere with little space. I hope that you'll find the associated burning sensation to be as satisfying as I do.

- Begin by locating a flat surface to stand and position your feet hip-width apart.
- Place the middle portion of the resistance band securely under your feet while ensuring that there is an even distribution of tension on both sides.
- While keeping your elbows tucked in at your sides, initiate the motion by simultaneously curling the resistance band handles upward to your shoulders.
- Gently return the handles all the way down to the starting position.
- Repeat.

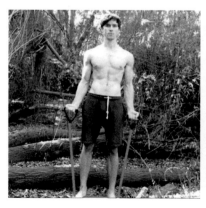
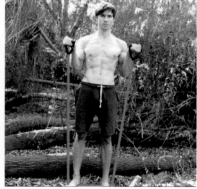

## *Exercise #4: Standing Calf Raise*

This super convenient callisthenic exercise exhausts the calves and can be done anywhere without any equipment. It is commonly performed while balancing the feet on a step in order to reach the full range of motion. However, I almost always do it on a flat surface and (in my opinion) it's just as effective. Step or no step, I think you'll reach similar gains.

- Begin by locating a firm and flat surface.
- While maintaining good posture in the standing position, place your feet hip-width apart, arms at your side, with abs pulled inward. Feel free to use an object (such as a tree) to gently place your hands against for added support. I prefer not to use added support, as this exercise can also help to improve balance.
- Start the motion by simultaneously raising the heels as high off the ground as they can go, until you are on your tiptoes.
- Gently return your heels to the ground before exploding back upward.
- Repeat.

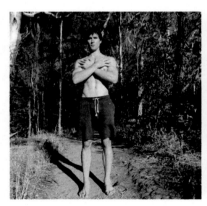 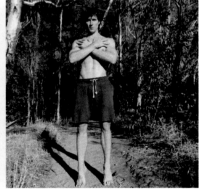

# Exercise #5: The Basic Crunch

The basic crunch is one of the most common and most effective exercises for improving strength and increasing definition within the abdominal muscles. It can be performed nearly anywhere as long as it is done on a supportive and comfortable surface. However, I think it's important to note that it should be temporarily avoided if you're currently experiencing any sort of pain within the lower back or neck regions, as the motion can further aggravate any existing injury.

- Begin by locating a flat and comfortable surface. I usually prefer a patch of a grass but a rolled-out yoga mat should do just fine.
- Lie down on your back and position your knees so that the angle between your hamstrings and calves is about 90 degrees. Position your thumbs so that they're in contact with the back of your ears (maintain this placement of the finger tips without using your hands for support of the head). Hold your elbows out toward your sides while rounding them slightly inward.
- Initiate the motion by curling your chest upward (elevating the shoulder blades from the ground), as if attempting to connect your face to the sky, keeping your eyes focused straight up to the clouds or to the ceiling. Pause for a moment before gently returning to the starting position.
- Repeat.

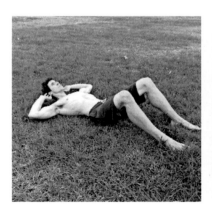
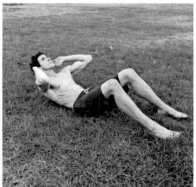

# Interval Circuit #3 (Friday)

Interval circuit #3 targets the triceps, shoulders, hamstrings, glutes, and core muscles. It is meant to be performed 48 hours after interval circuit #2. By completing this routine on Friday, you will allow your body enough time to properly recover before diving back into interval circuit #1 on Monday.

This circuit includes the following exercises:
   1) Resistance band overhead triceps extension - 20 reps
   2) Donkey kick - 60 reps (30 reps for each side)
   3) Resistance band lateral raise - 20 reps
   4) Short bridge - 30 reps
   5) Crunchy frog - 20 reps
— Rest for 60 seconds, then repeat the circuit.

- Have a stopwatch on hand (a smart phone works quite well).
- Repeat the circuit three times.
- Perform the first cycle with the lightest resistance band, second cycle with the middleweight band, and third cycle with heavyweight band.

# Exercise #1: Resistance Band Overhead Tricep Extension

This exercise is one of my favorites because of its effectiveness to carve and tone the arms. Exhausting the triceps with an isolation technique not only improves definition within the arm; it strengthens the upper body for all pushing motions where the chest and shoulders are involved.

- Begin by locating a sturdy object to sit on. Position your feet hip-width apart and place the middle of the resistance band under the souls of your shoes. Ensure that there is an even distribution of tension on both sides of the band.
- Grasp the handles behind your head with your palms facing upward. Position your elbows so that they are pointing outward in front of you and maintaining an even level with your head.
- Start the motion by pushing your forearms upward (while keeping the rest of the body stationary) until the arms are straight.
- Gently return to the starting position.
- Repeat.

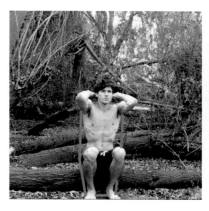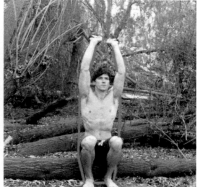

Braeden Baade

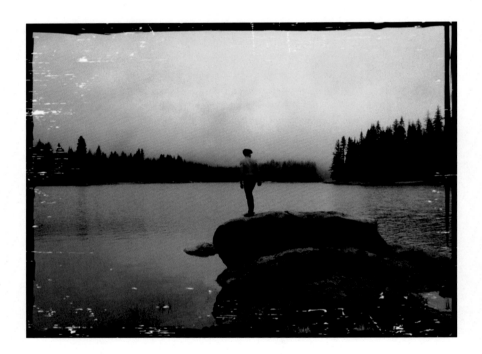

# Exercise #2: The Donkey Kick

This beginner level calisthenics exercise is a highly effective one for toning the hamstrings and glutes. It can be performed literally anywhere as long as there is a flat and comfortable enough surface available to support the knees and palms.

- Begin by locating a flat and supportive surface. I prefer to use a patch of grass but a yoga mat works just fine. Position your body so you are on your hands and knees. Ensure there is a 90-degree angle between your hamstrings and calves, and that your torso is parallel with the ground below.
- Initiate the motion by flexing your right foot and lifting your right leg until your knee becomes parallel with your right hip.
- Gently return to the starting position without allowing your right knee to touch the ground.
- After completing the reps with your right foot, repeat the exercise with the left foot.

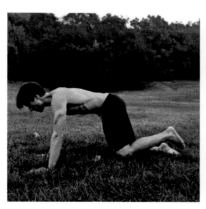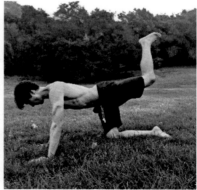

# Exercise #3: Resistance Band Lateral Raise

This resistance band exercise targets the deltoids (shoulders) and is excellent for adding definition between the shoulders and arms, as well as between the shoulders and traps (the back muscles that are connected to the neck).

- Begin by locating a flat and sturdy surface. Position your feet together and place them on the middle of the resistance band while ensuring that there is a balanced distribution of tension on both sides of the band.
- With palms facing inward toward your thighs, grasp the resistance band handles. Maintain a slight bend in your elbows throughout the exercise.
- To initiate the motion, lift your arms out from your sides until your hands are level with your shoulders. Briefly pause before gently lowering your arms to the starting position.
- Repeat.

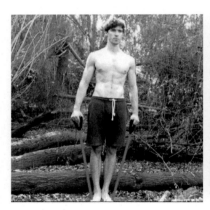 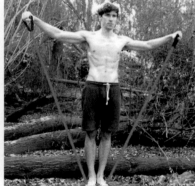

# Exercise #4: The Short Bridge

This beginner-level callisthenic exercise is not only convenient and easy to do, it's one of the best techniques for keeping your glutes and lower back in tiptop shape. Since the gluteus maximus (the butt) is the largest muscle in the human body, it's no mystery as to why it should be conditioned on a regular basis.

- Begin by locating a flat, sturdy, and comfortable surface to lie on your back.
- Position your feet to create a 90-degree bend in the knees. Place the arms loosely near the body or wherever they feel comfortable.
- To initiate the motion, raise your pelvis in the air until it can't go any further. Remember to pause momentarily while squeezing your glutes.
- Gently return to the starting position.
- Repeat.

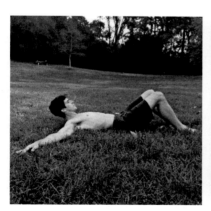 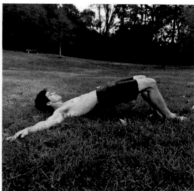

# Exercise #5: The Crunchy Frog

The crunchy frog is another one of my favorite calisthenics exercises for carving and strengthening the abdominal muscles. It's also quite advantageous to execute immediately after the previous exercise (the short bridge) as they combine to exhaust the core within an extended range of motion.

- Begin by locating a flat and sturdy surface to sit on.
- Set your body in a V-like position with arms at your sides to help with balance. Your back should be positioned about 45 degrees from the ground.
- To begin the motion, retract your knees toward your chest. Remember to flex the abdominal muscles and keep your feet off the ground through the duration of the exercise.
- Gently return to the starting position.
- Repeat.

NOTE: This exercise is also excellent for improving balance.

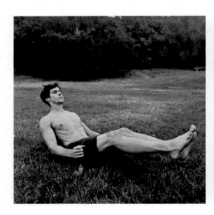 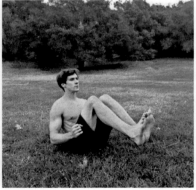

# The *Nature Physique* Isolation Routines

Given that you've now warmed your body up to resistance training with the previous interval routines, it's now time to further shock and develop the muscles by switching to a program of isolation techniques. The point of an isolation exercise is to target specific areas of specific muscles. As satisfying as these exercises can be, it's important to remember that it's almost impossible to work only one muscle at any given time. Even though you may feel the burn (lactic acid buildup) in a specific area during a movement, there are still plenty of other muscles that are tuning in as stabilizers to aid in controlling that motion. The isolation routines consist of exhausting one muscle group per day.

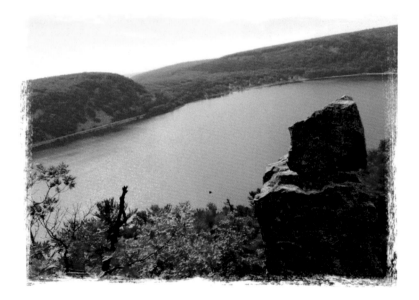

# Isolation Day 1: Chest (Monday)

For isolation day #1 we will focus on exhausting the various areas of the chest. Prominent and strong pectorals are one of the most desirable attributes for the human physique so it's crucial we engage each section of those large muscles. Day #1 is composed of a variety of both calisthenics (body weight exercises) and resistance band exercises to create a convenient and productive workout routine.

This routine includes the following exercises:
1) Regular push up - 2 sets (20 reps)
2) Resistance band chest fly - 2 sets (30 reps)
3) Incline push up - 2 sets (20 reps)
4) Resistance band decline chest fly - 2 sets (30 reps)
5) Wide grip push up - 2 sets (15 reps)

- Perform each set with 45 seconds of rest between each exercise (use a stopwatch).
- Remember that the repetition amounts that are listed above only serve as a general base. Feel free to increase or decrease the repetition amount to cater to your current comfort and fitness level; but always ensure that you're feeling the burn.
- Start the resistance band exercises using the lighter band and then progress to the middle band or heavy band. Always experiment with the number of repetitions to further shock your muscles.

# Exercise #1: The Regular Push Up

- Begin by locating a flat and sturdy surface.
- After getting down on the ground, position your hands so that they are just a tad bit wider than shoulder-width. You can position your hands in whatever way feels most supportive and comfortable. As for the positioning of my feet, I like to place them about hip-width apart as this feels most comfortable and encourages better form.
- To ensure that your body is properly aligned through the duration of the exercise, it helps to flex your abs, as well as your butt.
- To initiate the motion, lower your body toward the ground until your elbows create a 90-degree angle, then explode back up to the starting position.
- Repeat.

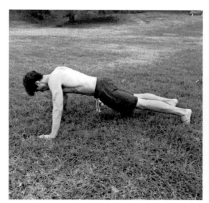
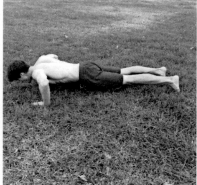

# Exercise #2: Resistance Band Chest Fly

- Begin by locating a tree (or something sturdy) to wrap the center of the resistance band around to create an anchor.
- With your back facing the tree, grasp a band handle in each hand. Position your arms so that they are spread out to your sides just below shoulder level. Place one foot out in front of the other while maintaining a slight bend in the knees through the duration of the exercise.
- To initiate the motion, bring your hands together outward and in front of your body while keeping a tiny bend in your elbows. Remember to squeeze your chest at the end of the repetition.
- Gently return to the starting position.
- Repeat.

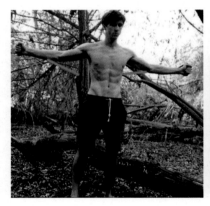
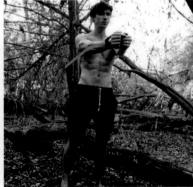

# Exercise #3: Incline Push Up

- Begin by locating a platform (such as a boulder, fallen tree, picnic bench, etc.) that's knee-level in height.
- Rest your hands on the platform at the same angle that felt comfortable with the regular push up and ensure that they're a little bit wider than shoulder-width apart. Keep your feet extended far enough out on the ground so that your body creates the same straight line as in the regular push up.
- Carefully lower your body until your chest just barely touches the edge of the platform, and then explode back upward to the starting position.
- Repeat.

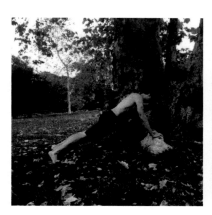 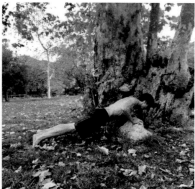

# Exercise #4: Resistance Band Decline Chest Fly

- Begin by locating a sturdy tree branch to anchor the center of the resistance band from above. Depending on the height of the available branch, you can choose to perform this exercise while either standing or kneeling.
- Once the band is securely anchored, grasp each handle with your arms spread out from your sides, at a level just below the shoulders, and with a slight bend in the elbows. Position your torso so that your chest is slightly angled toward the ground.
- Start the motion by bringing both arms down toward the ground until your hands meet in front of your chest. Take a brief pause while mindfully squeezing your pectorals before gently returning the arms to the starting position.
- Repeat.

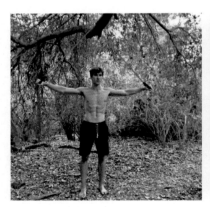 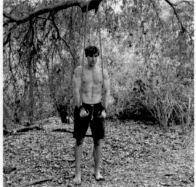

# Exercise #5: Wide Grip Push Up

- Begin by locating a flat and sturdy surface.
- Position your body in a similar manner as to how you'd perform the regular push up. Place your hands and feet so that they are both wider than shoulder-width. Remember to have your body maintain a straight line from your back to your feet through the duration of the exercise.
- Initiate the motion by slowly lowering your chest until it's just barely above the ground. Flex your pectoral and abdominal muscles as you explode back upward to the starting position.
- Repeat.

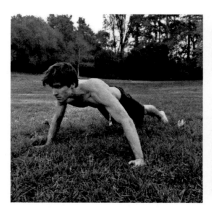
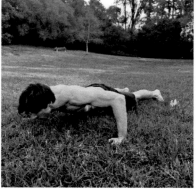

# Isolation Day 2: Biceps (Tuesday)

For isolation day #2 we will focus on exhausting the different areas of the biceps. This routine consists of a variety of resistance band pulling motions to trigger improvement in definition, strength, and endurance within the frontal portion of the upper-arms, as well as the forearms.

This routine includes the following exercises:
1) Resistance band standing bicep curl - 2 sets (30 reps)
2) Resistance band one arm concentration curl - 2 sets (20 reps each side)
3) Resistance band cross-body hammer curl - 2 sets (20 reps each side)
4) Resistance band reverse bicep curl - 2 sets (30 reps)

- Perform each set with 45 seconds of rest between each exercise (use a stopwatch).
- Remember that the repetition amounts that are listed above only serve as a general base. Feel free to increase or decrease the repetition amount to cater to your current comfort and fitness level; but always ensure that you're feeling the burn.
- Start the resistance band exercises using the lighter band and then progress to the middle band or heavy band. Always experiment with the number of repetitions to further shock your muscles.

# Exercise #1: Resistance Band Standing Bicep Curl

- Begin by locating a flat surface to stand and position your feet hip-width apart.
- Place the middle portion of the resistance band securely under your feet while ensuring that there is an even distribution of tension on both sides.
- While keeping your elbows tucked in at your sides, initiate the motion by simultaneously curling the resistance band handles upward to your shoulders.
- Gently return the handles all the way down to the starting position.
- Repeat.

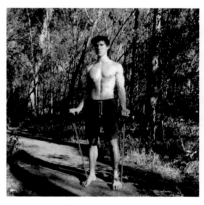 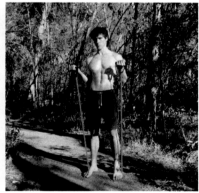

## Exercise #2: Resistance Band One Arm Concentration Curl

- Begin by locating a flat and sturdy surface to stand.
- Position your feet on top of the center of the resistance band, place your right elbow on your right thigh, while grasping one handle with your right hand. Lean your torso a tiny bit forward so that there is a slight bend in your back.
- To initiate the motion, maintain a stillness throughout your body while curling only your forearm upward as far as it can go, then gently lower your forearm back to the starting position.
- Repeat for the recommended amount of repetitions before switching to your left side.

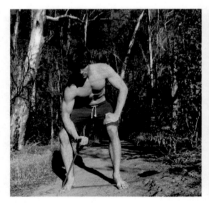 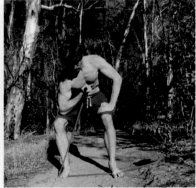

# Exercise #3: Resistance Band Cross-Body Hammer Curl

- Begin by locating a flat and sturdy surface to stand.
- Place the middle of the resistance band under your feet just as you would while performing the standing bicep curl. Position your feet hip-width apart and maintain a strong, erect posture. Grip a band handle in each hand while both palms face inward toward your body. Your palms should stay directed inward throughout the duration of the exercise.
- Begin the motion by curling your right forearm across your body and up toward your left shoulder. Flex the bicep while pausing for a moment before gently returning your right forearm to the starting position. Now mirror the motion by curling your left forearm up toward your right shoulder.
- Alternate sides until the designated repetitions are completed.

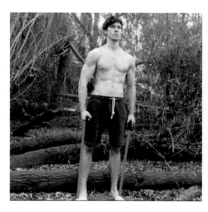
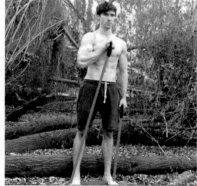

## *Exercise #4: Resistance Band Reverse Bicep Curl*

- Begin by locating a flat and sturdy surface to stand.
- Identical to the standing bicep curl, stand fully erect with your feet together and placed on the center of the resistance band. Position your upper arms so that they're touching your oblique muscles and hold them there for the duration of the exercise. Grip a band handle in each hand with your palms facing toward the ground (opposite to the regular standing bicep curl).
- To begin the motion, curl your forearms upward to the point where your knuckles nearly contact your shoulders, then flex the biceps momentarily before gently lowering back down to the starting position.
- Repeat.

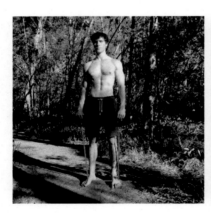 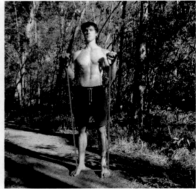

# Isolation Day 3: Legs (Wednesday)

Isolation day #3 combines resistance band and calisthenics exercises to improve vascularity, strength, and endurance of the various leg and lower-body muscles. Performing a leg routine on the third day has an added benefit as it allows for added upper-body recovery time.

This routine includes the following exercises:
1) Resistance band squat - 2 sets (30 reps)
2) Fire hydrant - 2 sets on each side (30 reps)
3) Tree sit - 2 sets (hold for 30 seconds)
4) Good morning - 2 sets (30 reps)
5) Single leg calf raise - 2 sets on each side (30 reps)

- Perform each set with 45 seconds between each exercise (use a stopwatch).
- Remember that the repetition amounts that are listed above only serve as a general base. Feel free to increase or decrease the repetition amount to cater to your current comfort and fitness level; but always ensure that you're feeling the burn.
- Start the resistance band exercises using the lighter band and then progress to the middle band or heavy band. Always experiment with the number of repetitions to further shock your muscles.

# *Exercise #1: Resistance Band Squat*

- Begin by locating a flat and sturdy surface to stand.
- Place the center of the resistance band under your feet and position your feet so that they are hip-width apart. Grip the band handles so that they're stretched to shoulder-level and resting in front of your arms. Make sure that there is an even distribution of tension on both sides of your body.
- To begin the motion, squat down until your butt is nearly leveled with your knees, then gently push back up to the starting position. Remember to maintain a straight back and to also focus all your weight onto your heels through the duration of the exercise.
- Repeat.

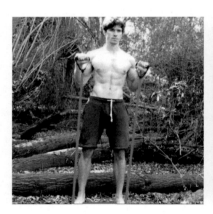
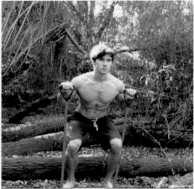

# Exercise #2: The Fire Hydrant

- Begin by locating a comfortable and sturdy surface.
- Rest your body onto your hands and knees. To ensure good form, place your hands directly below your shoulders and spread your knees to shoulder-width apart.
- To initiate the motion, lift your right knee and right foot outward to the side of your body until it is nearly level with your right glute. Flex your right glute momentarily before lowering to the starting position.
- Repeat until you reach the designated number of repetitions and then perform the exercise on your left side.

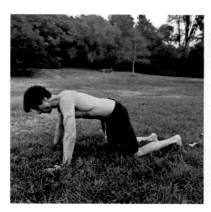
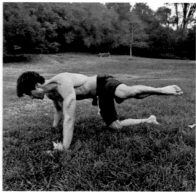

# Exercise #3: The Tree Sit

- Begin by locating a straight, thick, and sturdy tree (or select a spot on the wall if you're performing your exercise routine while indoors).
- Rest your back against the tree and lower your body to the point where a 90-degree angle is formed at the knees. Position your feet so that they're shoulder-width apart. A good strategy to ensure that your positioning is correct is to check that your feet are directly below your knees.
- Have a stop-watch within reach and initiate the exercise as soon as you are in the correct stance. Hold your body in place for 30 seconds or until you feel a deep burn in your legs.
- Rest for 30 seconds and then repeat.

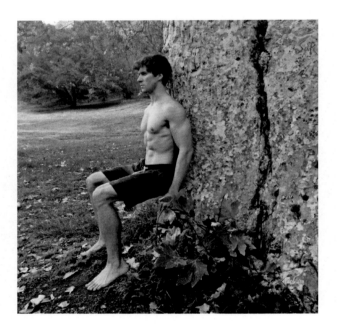

# Exercise #4: The Good Morning

- Begin by locating a flat and sturdy surface to stand.
- Position your feet so that they're hip-width apart. Stand fully erect as you gently place your hands on the back of your head and angle your elbows outward to the sides.
- To begin the motion, flex your abs and lean your butt backward as you lower your torso until it is nearly parallel with the ground. Remember to maintain a slight bend in the knees as you lower the torso. Carefully return to the starting position.
- Repeat.

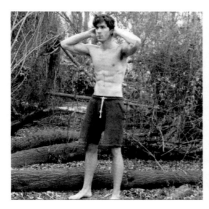 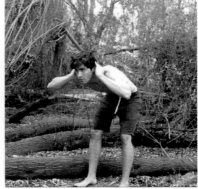

# Exercise #5: The Single Leg Calf Raise

- Begin by locating a flat and sturdy spot on the ground near an object for hand-support such as a tree or a wall.
- Stand erect close enough to the tree/wall so that you can lightly rest your fingertips against it. Once you are comfortable, lift your left foot off the ground so that all your weight is distributed onto your right foot and hold it there until you reach the designated number of repetitions.
- To initiate the motion, raise your right heel upward as far as it can go and then gently lower it until it contacts the ground.
- Repeat for the designated number of reps before performing the mirrored motion with the left foot.

- NOTE: For an added challenge, perform the exercise while letting your hands hang loosely at your sides. This will help to further improve balance.

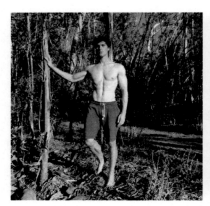 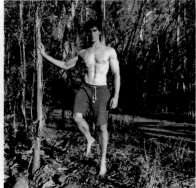

# Isolation Day 4: Triceps (Thursday)

Isolation day #4 combines calisthenics and resistance band exercises to work all angles of the triceps, improving definition, strength, and endurance. The triceps play a significant role with most upper-body pushing motions so it's essential to give them adequate attention.

This routine includes the following exercises:
1) Rock dip - 2 sets (20 reps)
2) Resistance band triceps pushdown - 2 sets (20 reps)
3) Diamond push up - 2 sets (20 reps)
4) Resistance band one arm overhead triceps extension - 2 sets each side (20 reps)

- Perform each set with 45 seconds rest in between each exercise (use a stopwatch).
- Remember that the repetition amount listed above only serves as a general base. Feel free to increase or decrease the repetition amount to your comfort and current fitness level, but always ensure that you're feeling the burn.
- Start the resistance band exercises using the lighter band and then progress to the middle band or heavy band. Always experiment to your liking to further shock your muscles.

# *Exercise #1: The Rock Dip*

- Begin by locating either a sturdy rock, park bench, or chair (if indoors).
- Stand with your back turned toward the rock, lower your body, anchor your hands on the edge, and bend your knees to about 90 degrees as if you we're sitting in a chair.
- To begin the motion, slowly lower your body until your elbows are nearly bent to a 90-degree angle (as you shouldn't go any lower to avoid risking injury).
- Carefully push upward to the starting position.
- Repeat.

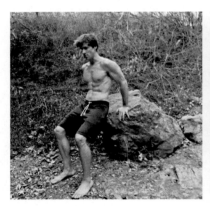 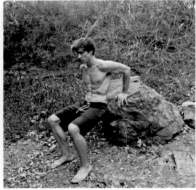

# Exercise #2: The Resistance Band Tricep Pushdown

- Begin by locating a tree that is equipped with a sturdy branch above head-height.
- Toss the resistance band over the branch so that the center is anchored with an even distribution of tension on both sides of the band. Grasp a handle in each hand (palms facing toward the ground), with elbows locked at your sides, and feet positioned hip-width apart. Maintain this stance throughout the duration of the exercise.
- Initiate the motion by pushing your forearms downward until your elbows nearly straighten, flex your triceps, then gently return to the starting position.
- Repeat.

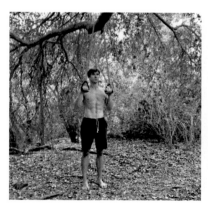 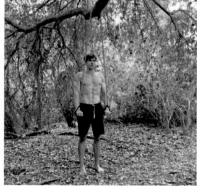

# Exercise #3: The Diamond Push Up

- Begin by locating a flat and supportive surface to get down into the regular push up position.
- Once you are comfortable on the ground, move your hands together to the point where your index fingers and thumbs form a diamond shape directly below your chest. Spread your feet so that they are hip-with apart.
- To begin the motion, carefully lower your body, briefly contacting the ground, then push back up until your arms are fully extended.
- Repeat.

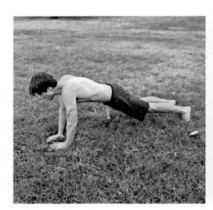 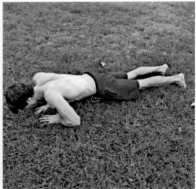

# Exercise #4: Resistance Band One Arm Overhead Tricep Extension

- Begin by locating a flat and sturdy surface to stand on.
- Stand hip-width apart and place one end of the resistance band under your feet and grip the other end with your right hand. Raise your right arm upward to the point where your right elbow is near full extension and your right palm is facing forward.
- To initiate the motion, carefully lower your right forearm until it nearly touches the bicep, all while maintaining a stillness throughout the rest of your body.
- Complete the designated number of repetitions before mirroring the exercise with your left arm.

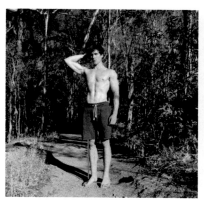 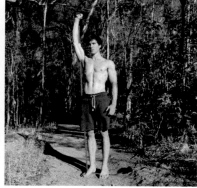

# Isolation Day 5: Back (Friday)

Isolation day #5 consists of both resistance band and calisthenics exercises to exhaust the various muscles of the upper and lower back. The back muscles play a large role not only in the upper body pulling motions, but also in stabilization with nearly every exercise.

This routine includes the following exercises:
1) Regular grip pull up - 2 sets (10 reps)
2) Resistance band standing row - 2 sets (30 reps)
3) Chin up - 2 sets (10 reps)
4) Resistance band shrug - 2 sets (50 reps)
5) Superman - 2 sets (10 reps)

- Perform each set with 45 seconds rest in between each exercise (use a stopwatch).
- Remember that the repetition amounts that are listed above only serve as a general base. Feel free to increase or decrease the repetition amount to cater to your current comfort and fitness level; but always ensure that you're feeling the burn.
- Start the resistance band exercises using the lighter band and then progress to the middle band or heavy band. Always experiment with the number of repetitions to further shock your muscles.

# Exercise #1: Regular Grip Pull Up

- Begin by locating a horizontal and sturdy tree branch that is within overhead reaching distance.
- Grip the branch with both hands, palms facing forward, and spread them a bit wider than shoulder-width. Let yourself hang loosely from the branch with locked elbows.
- To initiate the motion, tighten your abs and retract the shoulders as you pull your body up toward the branch until your elbows are nearly touching your oblique muscles; momentarily pause while flexing your back, then carefully lower your body to the starting position.
- Repeat.

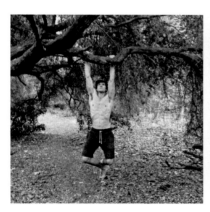
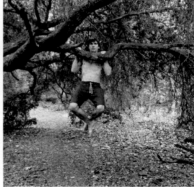

# Exercise #2: The Resistance Band Standing Row

- Begin by locating a sturdy tree to anchor the center of the resistance band.
- Stand facing the tree with about four feet of space in between and anchor the band so that it's just below chest-level. Position your feet so that they're hip-width apart, and grasp the handles with palms facing downward. Make sure to check that there is an even distribution of tension on both sides of the resistance band. Position your elbows at a height of just below shoulder level and maintain this throughout the duration of the exercise.
- To begin the motion, pull the handles inward until they nearly touch your chest and squeeze your back momentarily before gently returning to the starting position.
- Repeat.

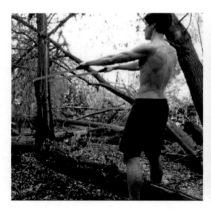 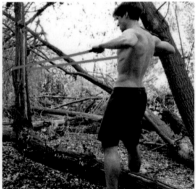

# Exercise #3: The Chin Up

- Begin by locating a horizontal and sturdy tree branch that is within overhead reaching distance.
- Grip the branch with both hands, palms facing toward your chest, and spread them shoulder-width apart.
- To begin the motion, pull your body upward to the point where your chin is level with or slightly above the branch, and elbows are at your sides. Momentarily squeeze your back muscles before gently lowering your body to the starting position.
- Repeat.

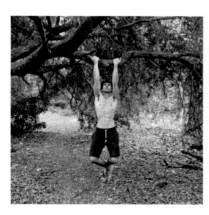
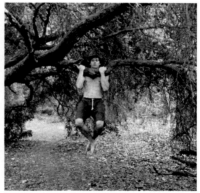

# Exercise #4: The Resistance Band Shrug

- Begin by locating a flat and sturdy surface to stand.
- Position your feet so that they are hip-width apart and place the center of the resistance band underneath. Grasp a handle in each hand while ensuring that there is an even distribution of resistance on both sides of the band. Slightly tilt your torso forward to fully engage the upper back muscles (traps). Let your arms hang loosely at your sides.
- To initiate the motion, shrug the shoulders upward toward your ears, and then backward in a semicircular motion. Make sure to momentarily pause at the peak of the motion before returning to the starting position.
- Repeat.

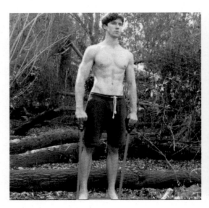 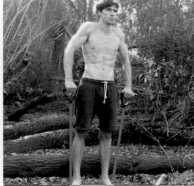

# Exercise #5: The Superman

- Begin by locating a flat and comfortable surface.
- Position your body so that you are lying flat on your stomach with your arms and legs fully extended outward, palms facing down toward the ground; ensure that your elbows and knees are completely straight.
- To begin the motion, simultaneously raise your arms and legs off the ground while placing all of your weight onto your core. Squeeze your lower back and butt while holding the position for two seconds; gently return to the starting position.
- Repeat.

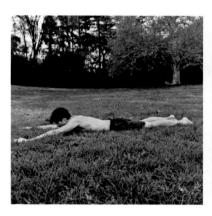 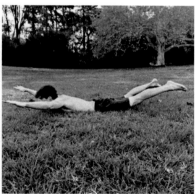

# Isolation Day 6: Shoulders (Saturday)

Isolation day #6 consists of multiple resistance band and calisthenics exercises in order to target the various shoulder muscles. Strong shoulders help to increase overall upper-body strength, stabilization, and posture.

This routine includes the following exercises:
1) Resistance band upright row - 2 sets (20 reps)
2) Resistance band shoulder press - 2 sets (20 reps)
3) Resistance band lateral raise - 2 sets (20 reps)
4) Resistance band front raise - 2 sets (20 reps)

- Perform each set with 45 seconds rest in between each exercise (use a stopwatch).
- Remember that the repetition amounts that are listed above only serve as a general base. Feel free to increase or decrease the repetition amount to cater to your current comfort and fitness level; but always ensure that you're feeling the burn.
- Start the resistance band exercises using the lighter band and then progress to the middle band or heavy band. Always experiment with the number of repetitions in order to further shock your muscles.

# Exercise #4: Resistance Band Upright Row

- Begin by locating a flat surface.
- Form a stance that is shoulder-width apart. Place the middle of the resistance band carefully under your feet. Make sure the band's tension feels balanced on both sides of your body.
- While maintaining good posture, raise your hands until they nearly meet your collarbone. For optimal form, attempt to consistently raise the elbows slightly higher than the hands. This will trigger more of the muscle's range of motion.
- Gently lower your arms all the way down to the starting point before carefully exploding back upward.
- Repeat.

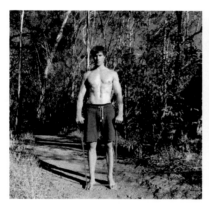 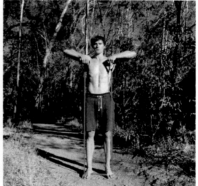

## Exercise #2: The Resistance Band Shoulder Press

- Begin by locating a flat and sturdy spot on the ground.
- Position your feet together and place the center of the resistance band underneath while ensuring that there is an even distribution of tension on both sides. Grasp a handle in each hand and face the palms forward with the band in front of your elbows and forearms.
- To begin the motion, press your arms straight up into the air until they are near full extension, then gently lower the elbows back to the starting position.
- Repeat.

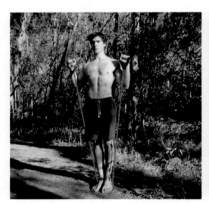 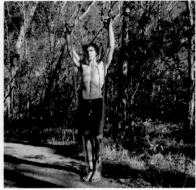

# Exercise #3: Resistance Band Lateral Raise

- Begin by locating a flat and sturdy surface to stand.
- Position your feet together and place the center of the resistance band underneath your feet while ensuring that there is an even distribution of tension on either side of the band. Grip a band handle with each hand (palms facings inward toward your hips) and allow your arms to hang loosely at your sides.
- To initiate the motion, simultaneously raise both arms outward until your body forms a T-shape. Gently lower your arms back to the starting position. Make sure to maintain a slight bend in the elbows throughout the duration of the exercise.
- Repeat.

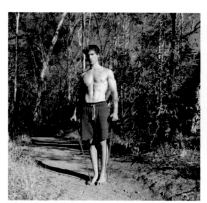
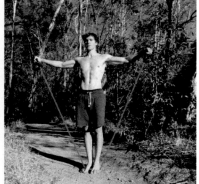

# Exercise #4: Resistance Band Front Raise

- Begin by locating a flat and sturdy spot on the ground.
- Position your feet so that they are spread hip-width apart. Place the center of the resistance band underneath your feet while double-checking that there is an even amount of tension on both sides. With your arms hanging loosely at your sides, grip a handle in each hand and turn your wrists so that your palms face backward.
- To begin the motion, simultaneously lift both arms forward and upward until your hands are level with your shoulders. Maintain a slight bend within the elbows throughout the duration of the exercise.
- Repeat.

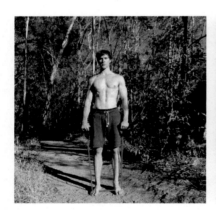
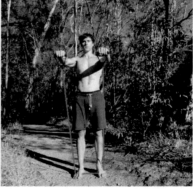

# Isolation Day 7: Core (Sunday)

Isolation day #7 combines resistance band and calisthenics exercises to improve definition, strength, and endurance of the abdominal muscles. It serves us well to dedicate an entire routine to the development of the core muscles so that we reduce the risk of *half-assing* them or even neglecting them altogether.

This routine includes the following exercises:
1) Sit up - 2 sets (30 reps)
2) Lying leg raise - 2 sets (20 reps)
3) Basic crunch - 2 sets (20 reps)
4) Resistance band kneeling crunch - 2 sets (20 reps)
5) Resistance band oblique side bend - 2 sets on each side (30 reps)

- Perform each set with 45 seconds in between each exercise (use a stopwatch).
- Remember that the repetition amounts that are listed above only serve as a general base. Feel free to increase or decrease the repetition amount to cater to your current comfort and fitness level; but always ensure that you're feeling the burn.
- Start the resistance band exercises using the lighter band and then progress to the middle band or heavy band. Always experiment with the number of repetitions to further shock your muscles.

# Exercise #1: The Sit Up

- Begin by locating a flat and comfortable patch on the ground.
- Lie down on your back with feet flat and knees bent to 90 degrees and position your hands across your chest.
- To initiate the motion, flex your abs while raising your torso toward your knees, then gently lower back to the starting position.
- Repeat.

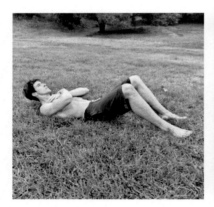
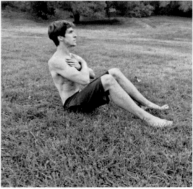

# Exercise #2: The Lying Leg Raise

- Begin by locating a flat and comfortable spot on the ground.
- Lie on your back, and position your arms outward at your sides with palms facing down. Place your feet together and extend your legs straight out.
- To begin the motion, simultaneously raise both legs until a 90 degree angle is formed between your upper and lower-body. Immediately lower to the point where heels are almost touching the ground, then explode back upward.
- Repeat.

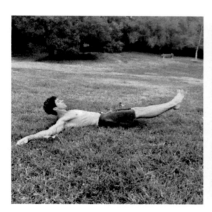
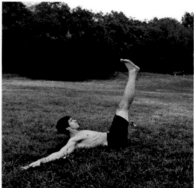

# *Exercise #3: The Basic Crunch*

- Begin by locating a flat and comfortable surface.
- Lie down on your back and position your knees so that the angle between your hamstrings and calves is about 90 degrees. Position your thumbs so that they're in contact with the back of your ears. Hold your elbows out toward your sides while rounding them slightly inward.
- Initiate the motion by curling your chest upward (elevating the shoulder blades from the ground), as if attempting to connect your face to the sky, keeping your eyes focused straight above to the clouds or to the ceiling. Pause for a moment before gently returning to the starting position.
- Repeat.

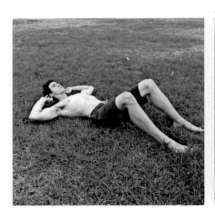 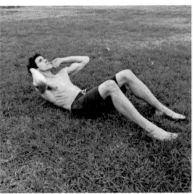

# Exercise #4: The Resistance Band Kneeling Crunch

- Begin by locating a low and sturdy tree branch to anchor the resistance band.
- Loop the center of the resistance band on top of the tree branch and make sure that there is an even distribution of tension on each side. Grasp the handles and kneel in front of the tree. Bend your elbows so that they face forward in front of your body at shoulder level.
- To initiate the motion, flex your abs as you lower your torso toward the ground. Make sure to arch your back as your elbows nearly connect with the ground. Carefully return your torso back to the starting position.
- Repeat.

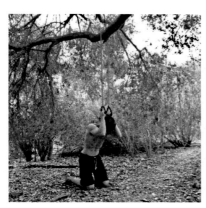
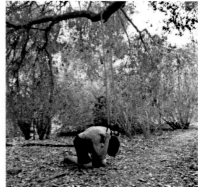

# Exercise #5: The Resistance Band Oblique Side Bend

- Begin by locating a flat patch on the ground to stand.
- Position the feet so that they are spread hip-width apart and place the center of the resistance band under your right foot. Squeeze both sides of the band (from knee level) together with your right hand while resting your left hand loosely at your side.
- To begin the motion, lean your torso toward your ride side before returning to the starting position.
- Complete the designated repetition amount before mirroring the exercise with your left hand.
- Repeat.

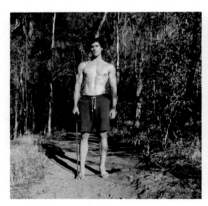 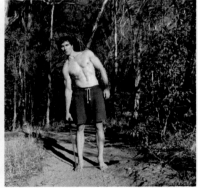

# The *Nature Physique* Superset Routine

The third and final phase of the *nature physique* routine is intended to take your progress to new heights. The intention of a "superset" is to exhaust multiple areas within the body to trigger further gains within a full range of motion (usually combining a pushing motion with a pulling motion within the same region). An example of a superset would be to perform one set of a triceps exercise and then immediately follow it up with a bicep exercise. Upon finishing the triceps exercise (pushing motion), the surrounding stabilizer muscles and tendons will be momentarily exhausted, therefore this is an excellent time to implement a bicep exercise (pulling motion) to further work those stabilizing muscles and tendons; think of it as killing three birds with one stone!

# Superset Day 1: Chest & Back (Monday)

For superset day #1 we will target the multiple areas of the chest, multiple areas of the back, as well as the surrounding, stabilizer muscle tissues that are fortunately caught in the middle. Day #1 is composed of various calisthenics and resistance band exercises. We will close out each routine with a core exercise.

This routine includes the following exercises:
1) Regular push up + resistance band standing row - 4 sets
    a.   (execute both exercises until exhaustion)
2) Resistance band chest fly + wide grip pull up - 4 sets
    a.   (execute both exercises until exhaustion)
3) Basic crunch + the superman - 4 sets
    a.   (execute both exercises until exhaustion)

- Have a stopwatch nearby and rest 90 seconds in between each superset.
- Start the resistance band exercises using the lighter band and then progress to the middle band or heavy band. Always experiment with the number of repetitions to further shock your muscles.

# Superset #1: Regular Pushup + Resistance Band Standing Row

- For this superset I recommend you begin by locating a sturdy tree, grounded pole, etc. and wrap the center of the resistance band around it so that it is readily available upon finishing your set of regular push-ups.
- It's best to perform the set of push-ups within proximity to your selected resistance band anchor in order to execute the superset with maximum efficiency.
- Rest for 90 seconds after executing each superset.
- Repeat.

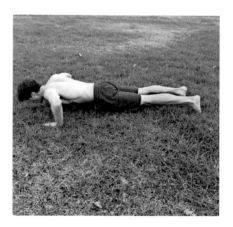

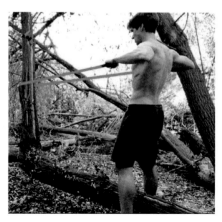

# Superset #2: Resistance Band Chest Fly + Wide Grip Pull Up

- Like the previous superset, it's crucial that you locate a sturdy branch or pull up bar that is near your resistance band anchor as this will help to reduce the passing of time in between the exercises.
- Rest for 90 seconds after executing each superset.
- Repeat.

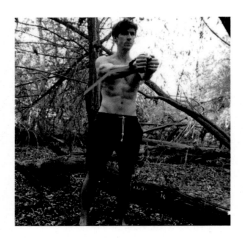

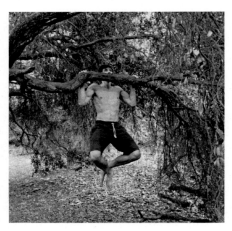

# Superset #3: Basic Crunch + The Superman

- Begin by locating a flat and sturdy surface that will enable you to comfortably lie on the ground.
- Perform the basic crunch until failure, then immediately turn over onto your stomach to perform the superman without any delay.
- Rest for 90 seconds after executing each superset.
- Repeat.

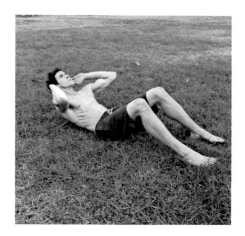

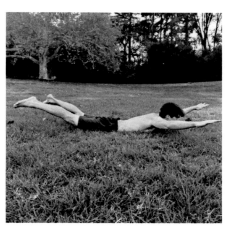

# Superset Day 2: Legs + Shoulders (Wednesday)

For superset day #2 we will focus on the various muscles of the legs, shoulders, along with the surrounding stabilizer-tissues and tendons. We will implement a series of both resistance band and callisthenic exercises. We will finish the routine with a core-based superset.

This routine includes the following exercises:
1) Resistance band shoulder press + prison squats - 4 sets
   a. (execute both exercises until exhaustion)
2) Resistance band front raise + standing calf raise - 4 sets
   a. (execute both exercises until exhaustion)
3) Regular sit up + the short bridge - 4 sets
   a. (execute both exercises until exhaustion)

- Have a stopwatch nearby and rest 90 seconds in between each superset.
- Start the resistance band exercises using the lighter band and then progress to the middle band or heavy band. Always experiment to your liking to further shock your muscles.

# Superset #1: Resistance Band Shoulder Press + Prison Squats

- Begin by locating a flat and sturdy spot on the ground.
- Perform the resistance band shoulder press, then toss the resistance band to the side and immediately begin the set of prison squats.
- Rest for 90 seconds after each superset.
- Repeat.

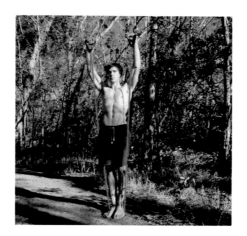

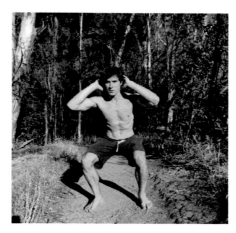

# Superset #2: Resistance Band Front Raise + Standing Calf Raise

- Begin by locating a flat and sturdy surface on the ground.
- After executing the resistance band front raise, immediately toss the resistance band aside and begin the standing calf raise.
- Rest for 90 seconds after each superset.
- Repeat.

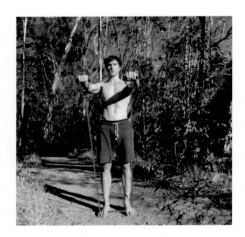

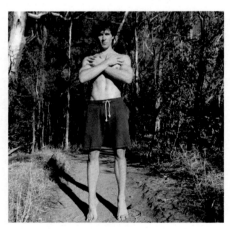

## Superset #3: Regular Sit Ups + Short Bridge

- Start by locating a flat, supportive, and comfortable area to lie down on the ground.
- After executing the regular sit ups, remain in that same position and immediately begin the short bridge.
- Rest for 90 seconds after each superset.
- Repeat.

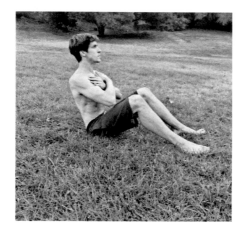

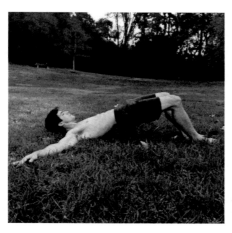

# Superset Day 3: Biceps + Triceps (Friday)

For superset day #3 we will target the primary muscles of the arms (biceps and triceps), as well as the surrounding stabilizer tissue and tendons. This routine combines a variety of callisthenic and resistance band exercises. We will then finish the routine with a core-based superset.

This routine includes the following exercises:
1) Chin up + resistance band triceps pushdown - 4 sets
    a. (execute both exercises until exhaustion)
2) Resistance band standing bicep curl + chair dip - 4 sets
    a. (execute both exercises until exhaustion)
3) Lying leg raise + crunchy frog - 4 sets
    a. (execute both exercises until exhaustion)

- Have a stopwatch nearby and rest 90 seconds in between each superset.
- Start the resistance band exercises using the lighter band and then progress to the middle band or heavy band. Always experiment with the number of repetitions to further shock your muscles.

# Superset #1: Chin Up + Resistance Band Triceps Pushdown

- Begin by locating a sturdy and over-head tree branch. The designated branch will serve as a pull-up bar, as well as an anchor for the resistance band.
- Perform the chin-ups until exhaustion, then immediately place the center of the resistance band on the tree branch and begin the triceps pushdown until fatigue.
- Rest for 90 seconds after each superset.
- Repeat.

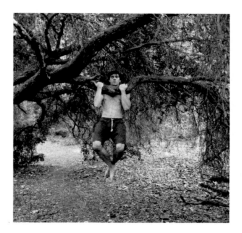

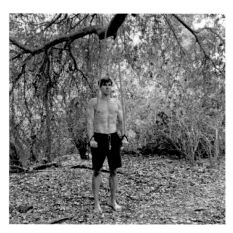

# Superset #2: Resistance Band Standing Bicep Curl + Rock Dip

- Start by locating a supportive object that is similar in height to the seat of a chair. This could be anything from a picnic bench to a boulder.
- Execute the resistance band standing bicep curl until exhaustion, toss the resistance band aside and immediately begin the chair dip exercise, also until exhaustion.
- Rest for 90 seconds after each superset.
- Repeat.

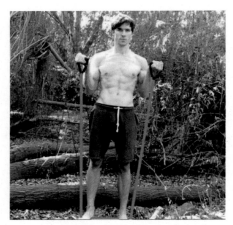

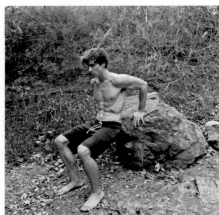

## Superset #3: Lying Leg Raise + Crunchy Frog

- Begin by locating a firm, flat, and comfortable spot on the ground.
- Gently lie down on your back, place your feet together and initiate the lying leg raise until exhaustion. When you've finished, position your weight onto your glutes and immediately perform the crunchy frog, also until exhaustion.
- Rest for 90 seconds after each superset.
- Repeat.

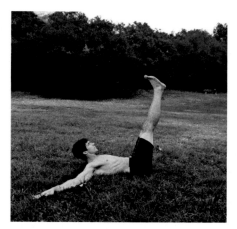

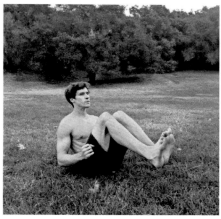

# Static Stretching: A Post-Workout Cool Down

To fully wrap up the exercise routine section, it's important I share a brief explanation as to why it is so much more beneficial (and safer) to engage in static stretching **AFTER** your workout rather than **BEFORE**. For those that aren't already aware, static stretching is done by stretching a muscle within a stationary and comfortable position, then holding that position for around 15 to 30 seconds. It's important to ensure that the designated stretch is executed with a challenging but not overly uncomfortable pose, as you don't want to risk pulling or tearing of the muscles.

One of my favorite analogies is to relate muscles to candy taffy; their elasticity is extremely similar in the sense that when muscle or taffy is at a warmer state, it allows for better manipulation, thus limiting chance of snapping or breaking and encouraging a wider range of motion.

The key to static stretching is to stretch the muscle beyond its normal range of motion, making for a more efficient post-workout recovery. People who stretch on a regular basis experience less tension, improved strength, quicker recovery, and reduced risk of muscle or tendon related injury.

# Final Note:
# The *Nature Physique* Is Within You

As the author, my greatest pleasure is to visualize my readers turning to this page with a new-found sense of enthusiasm and the inspiration to achieve an underlying greatness that has been patiently waiting to reveal itself to you. Your *nature physique* speaks the truth of the potential that was always within.

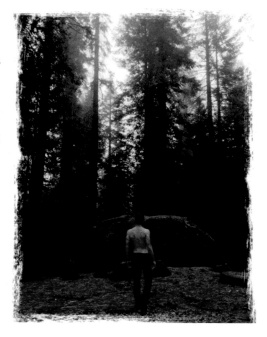

I encourage you to return to this text from time to time, not only to remind yourself of how simple and pleasurable a healthy lifestyle can be, but also as a strategy to fully absorb the knowledge contained within so that you can eventually make this information your own. I encourage you to pass these techniques onto someone close to you, or even an acquaintance that you believe could benefit from them.

Above all, maintain an attitude of gratitude, as this will undoubtedly aid you in your transcendence toward the greatness that nature intended for you.

Unleash your *nature physique.*

*Namaste.*

Braeden Baade

# Did You Enjoy *The Nature Physique?*

Before you continue your fitness journey, I'd very much like to say "thank you" for purchasing this guide.

I'm aware you had an endless variety of exercise books to select from, but you took a chance on my teachings.

Therefore, some huge thanks for purchasing this guide and for sticking with it all the way to the last page.

At this point, I'd like to ask you for a *tiny* favor. I'd be eternally grateful if you could head over to Amazon.com and write a quick review for *The Nature Physique.*

Your feedback will aid me as I continue to create Kindle books that you, as well as others, can benefit from. If you happened to find A LOT of value within the content, be sure to let me know :)

Last, but not least, feel free to visit my website at: http://www.NaturePhysiqueFitness.com from time to time, where you'll find new information on how to further improve your health and physique.

# Would You Like to Learn More?

You can learn quite a bit more on natural fitness within my other Kindle books. Guess what? I often run special promotions where I offer discounted (sometimes $0.99 or even **FREE**) books on Amazon.

A great way to find out about these offerings is to subscribe to my email list.

If you're often in search of new ways to challenge your body and improve your physique, I'd be honored if you would give my book *The Nature Physique: Easy Breezy Abs* a read. This book consists entirely of convenient, ab shredding workout routines; the best part is that all of them can be performed in under 15 minutes, at home... or in nature :)

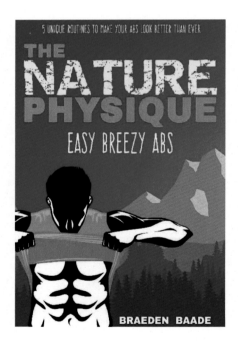

66623381R00075

Made in the USA
Middletown, DE
13 March 2018